TURNING BACK TO OURSELVES

In Praise of
Turning Back to Ourselves

"*Turning Back to Ourselves* is a wonderful guide for helping women develop their capacity to feel love and compassion for themselves. Providing a fine balance between spiritual wisdom, personal anecdotes, experiences with clients and practical exercises, the author does more than simply impart information—she writes in a way that makes you feel accompanied through it all. Written with humility and a reverence for the sacred, I highly recommend *Turning back to Ourselves* for spiritually minded women seeking reconciliation with themselves."

Jerry Lamagna Senior Faculty Member
at the AEDP Institute

"*Turning Back to Ourselves* offers an accessible integration of mindfulness practice and various therapeutic modalities. It incorporates personal stories of the author and various other women in clear and profound narratives of healing. It includes clear and concise explanations of mindfulness as well as very clear and valuable suggestions for practice and contemplation. This will be a valuable resource for many women as well as for teachers of mindfulness, practicing therapists, and spiritual directors."

Rabbi Sheila Peltz Weinberg,
author of *God Loves the Stranger*.

"In *Turning Back to Ourselves*, author Dalya Tamir insightfully, brilliantly lights a path for women that invites them to step out of the darkness of self–doubt and negativity into a new world, one in which they remember who they are, the power they have, and know their worth is not determined by the thoughts of others but by the fact that they are here in this world—they are a "light unto themselves. They are women."

Peaches Gillette, poet, preacher, and pastoral counselor,
author of *The Breadth of a Tree*.

"With her book *Turning Back to Ourselves*, Dalya Tamir offers a powerful, yet gentle and compassionate, journey to women of all ages and backgrounds who wish to (re)connect with themselves. By offering simple practices along the way, she takes us back to the truth of our heart and helps us embrace the depth of our sacred being. Truly transformative."

Séverine Orban, Ph.D. Meditation teacher and author of
Valentine Penrose – Le Pin sur la lune.

TURNING BACK TO OURSELVES

A Women's Guide to
Healing Self–Abandonment
and Loving Who We Are

DALYA TAMIR

Forewords by
James Baraz *and* Linda Graham

Copyright © 2024 by Dalya Tamir, LCSW
All rights reserved. This book or any portion thereof may not be reproduced or used in any manner whatsoever without written permission of the author.
First edition, February 2024.

This is a work of creative non-fiction. The stories of women offered in this book have been fictionalized. All names and identifying information have been changed. The women described, including members of the women's meditation circle, are compound characters. Anyone identified by name, including family members, has given full consent.

The information and advice contained in this book are based upon the personal and professional experiences of the author. They are not intended as a substitute for consulting with a healthcare professional for diagnosis or treatment. The author does not assume any guarantee and disclaims liability for any adverse results or consequences that result from suggestions or recommendations discussed in this book. All matters pertaining to your physical or mental health should be supervised by a healthcare professional.

Line on page 74 from "Widening Circles" by Rainer Maria Rilke
Line on page 80 from "St. Francis and the Sow" by Galway Kinnell
Line on page 174 from "After Apple Picking" by Robert Frost

Cover and interior book design by Bostjan Lisec, Slovenia.

ISBN 979-8-9898266-0-5 (Paperback.)
ISBN 979-8-9898266-1-2 (eBook.)
Library of Congress Control number: 2024900348

www.dalyatamir.com

Printed in the United States of America.

To the women who shaped my life:

My mother Adele

My mother-in-law Elsa

My aunt Gloria (Goggie)

My mentor Carol

Table of Contents

Foreword by James Baraz		XI
Foreword by Linda Graham		XIII
Introduction		XV
Chapter 1	Setting Out on the Journey Back to Ourselves: Understanding Self-Abandonment	1
Chapter 2	Bringing Our Attention to the Present: Turning Back with Mindfulness	25
Chapter 3	Taking Ourselves Back into Our Hearts: Turning Back with Compassion	51
Chapter 4	Releasing the Voice of Self-Judgment: Turning Back with Lovingkindness	73
Chapter 5	Coming Home to Our Bodies: Turning Back to Joy and Aliveness	99
Chapter 6	Living with Spaciousness: Turning Back to Center	133
Chapter 7	Befriending Our Lives: Abiding in the Wise and Compassionate Self	163
Acknowledgments		181
Resources		183
Recommended Reading		185
About the Author		187

Foreword by James Baraz

It may seem surprising for a man to be writing the foreword to a book on self–healing and self–actualization for women. Yet because patriarchal cultures have been the cause of women's pain and trauma through millennia, I welcomed with gratitude the opportunity to honor, acknowledge, and support the healing this book presents. *Turning Back to Ourselves* offers women a true pathway to heal the pain in their own lives and to free themselves from the constrictions of social conditioning in order to discover their intrinsic goodness.

As a longtime spiritual friend and mentor, I have shared with Dalya a love for the truth and the heart–opening power of meditation practice. This book is a testament to the wisdom and compassion which she has developed over a lifetime of deep introspection and generously supporting women to come fully into claiming who they are. The path she lays out in this book is an essential step in what in Buddhist practice is known as the journey of awakening.

As she points out, when we comprehend that each of us is an expression of life worthy of respect and love, we experience true happiness, joy, and well–being. Knowing that we belong and feeling a genuine connection to life aligns us with what is known as the Divine Feminine, that force of love and strength that naturally inclines toward the welfare of all.

In my work as a Buddhist meditation teacher, I have seen the power of practices such as mindfulness, self–compassion, and lovingkindness to help students move beyond the negative beliefs and conditioning that get in the way of that realization. *Turning Back to Ourselves* offers these time–tested tools in a brilliant, heartful and engaging way that invites the reader into a deep and lasting realization of their true nature. As we tenderly hold our habits of self–abandonment with compassion, we release the sense of contraction we may feel and open to spacious awareness and unconditional love. We not only understand but somatically realize our inherent goodness and divinity.

The power emerging in women as they turn back to themselves is one of the most important developments needed to transform our civilization. For this reason I would also encourage men to deepen their understanding of this cultural shift by reading this book. It gives me great pleasure to see *Turning Back to Ourselves* come to fruition. I know it will inspire and motivate many women to discover who they really are and to share their gifts with the world for the benefit of all. That is my wish for you and for everyone reading this book. May it be so.

James Baraz
January 2024

James Baraz is the co–founder of Spirit Rock Meditation Center, and the co–author of *Awakening Joy: Ten Steps to A Happier Life*.

Foreword by Linda Graham

Turning Back to Ourselves is an extraordinary gift for a wide range of readers. Dalya Tamir skillfully describes precisely how and why self-doubt, self-judgment, even self-hatred are so common in our culture, even inevitable in the condition of being human. And with great kindness and clarity, she provides a trustworthy path to the experience of inner goodness, worthiness, and inner peace so essential to abiding in health and wholeness.

Turning Back to Ourselves provides wisdom and practices for healing and transformation far more deeply than traditional self-help books. Dalya explores powerful practices of mindfulness, compassion, psychotherapy, centering the self and sharing with others – and makes the experiencing of them alive, vibrant, timely, and relevant.

In the exquisite storytelling and truth-telling of her own growing up and waking up and in the compassionate sharing of moments of self-recognition, self-acceptance, self-righting, and self-transformation in her women's circles, Tamir warmly invites the reader into the journey of self-discovery and self-flourishing.

I wish I'd had this book 30 years ago to hand to my clients finding their way through the dark and difficult, through openness and nurturing to a genuine experience of loving themselves and connecting to the sacred. The book is so well-structured, the honesty and transparency so compelling, the exercises so practical and doable. This is skillful guidance at its best.

Linda Graham
January 2024

Linda Graham, LMFT, is the author of *Bouncing Back: Rewiring Your Brain for Maximum Resilience and Well-Being*.

Introduction

Turning Back to Ourselves arose in response to the pain I have seen in women when they forget they are worthy of love, when they fall into patterns of judging and doubting themselves, when they place themselves outside the truth of their own hearts. In my work as a psychotherapist and in the meditation circles that I lead for women, I often hear: "I can love others, but I cannot love myself. I can forgive others but not myself. I can give to and care for others, but I find it hard to do the same for myself." This turning away from ourselves is what I call the pain of self-abandonment. Although layers of hurt and social conditioning may obscure our innate wisdom and hinder our ability to love ourselves, we all have the potential to turn back and hold ourselves with kindness. On this journey back to ourselves, we discover and reveal what we uniquely have to offer the world. *Turning Back to Ourselves* offers a path to guide us back home and a way to live with wisdom, compassion, and love.

My personal path of turning back to myself led me into the richness of Buddhist practice. Mindfulness showed me how to reconnect to myself, how to be aware without judgment of the thoughts and feelings arising in my mind, and how to respond with wisdom and discernment. Compassion taught me how to turn toward pain with caring attention. Lovingkindness taught me how to take myself back into my heart and then to extend my love to others.

This path back to ourselves is based in Buddhist practices that explicitly address who we are as women, a path that emphasizes compassion, connection, support, and safety; a path that embraces, not condemns, our female bodies, our sexuality, and our passion; a path that invites us to turn away from abandoning ourselves and return to being powerful, energetic, emotional, and thoughtful women. Whether you are involved in pursuing a career or dedicating your attention to raising a family, whether you are a young woman just discovering who you can be or a woman feeling the first signs of aging, this path invites you to turn back to yourself and rekindle a loving relationship with who you are.

Opening our hearts to ourselves takes a kind and heartful dedication to healing the ways in which we have been hurt. Maybe we did not feel loved as a child, or we struggled to find our place among our peers. Maybe we were told by our families or our culture that there was something wrong with us. Maybe we closed our hearts to ourselves as a result of overwhelming acts of physical, emotional, or sexual abuse. *Turning Back to Ourselves* is for those who, for any reason, have lost touch with their love for themselves.

As layers of defense that surround our hearts begin to soften, we learn to love ourselves and open to receive the love of others. With the safety and support of mindfulness, compassion, and lovingkindness, we gently and carefully allow that love in. Over time, as love deeply takes root in our heart, we take our place in the world with confidence and trust in ourselves.

Who and what is this "self" we are turning back to? According to Buddhist teachings, our sense of self—that which we call "me" or "I," the sense of who we are—is not an unchanging and separate entity but, rather, a flow of experience that arises moment by moment out of the causes and conditions that have brought us to this point in our life. When I talk about turning back to ourselves, I do not mean that are we returning to a specific image of ourselves or taking on an idealized image of who we think we should be, but rather we are recognizing ourselves as part of the river of experience that is the wholeness of life. Instead of regarding our "self" through the limiting habits of judgment and rejection, we open to each moment with curiosity, kindness, and love.

I offer this path as a fellow traveler, wishing to support women not only on their personal journey back to themselves but also to address the societal pressures that have had an impact on women through time and across cultures. In any exploration of how women turn away from themselves, this history must be taken into consideration and held in our awareness as we heal. And so, in *Turning Back to Ourselves,* I integrate the transformative power of feminist thinking with the wisdom of Buddhist teachings and insights from the world of psychotherapy.

We are living in an era when women are breaking through millennia-old patterns of repression, but the work continues. The dismantling of Roe v. Wade in 2023 may seem like a historical setback, but this apparent reversal of women's rights is only happening because we've moved so far forward. I continue to feel heartened when I speak to young women who have-experienced less gender discrimination than previous generations and are empowered to trust themselves as full participants and leaders in our world. I am inspired by women who will no longer be silent in the face of racial discrimination, sexual assault, and other forms of oppression. I am moved by women who are entering the political arena and by those who are breaking the boundaries of gender identity. Our inner work of turning back to ourselves and our work of social change are inseparable. By refusing to abandon ourselves, by holding ourselves in love no matter what we're facing, we are making both a personal and a political statement. In loving ourselves as women, we are speaking a language of inclusivity, equality, and worth. In finding our voices and speaking our truths, we are speaking up for ourselves as individuals and for all women.

We are in the midst of a revolution of awakening to difference and diversity of gender identity. I offer a wholehearted apology to gender nonconforming readers for any blind spots or inaccuracies in what I present in this book. As a white woman, I acknowledge the devastating impact of white privilege on Black, Indigenous, and People of Color (BIPOC) in our society, and I accept responsibility for ways I have participated in these forms of oppression. As we come to a deeper understanding of ourselves in light of these personal and societal pressures that have led to self-abandonment, our commitment to create a more open and just society grows.

The journey back to ourselves is unique for each of us. There is no set timeline or way it should evolve. I suggest reading this book slowly and carefully, listening to your inner responses to the words and stories. You may ask yourself: *What rings true to me? What is helpful? What is not? What brings a smile to my face? What brings tears? What questions arise?* Listen to your inner wisdom and call forth trust in yourself. Establishing a time and place to engage in daily meditation practice will also support that intention. Calming your mind through stillness of the body or through mindful awareness of movement in walking meditation will help you grow in self–awareness. And practicing lovingkindness will open you to recognizing your beauty and remembering that you are worthy of love. Joining with other women in meditation and reading *Turning Back to Ourselves* together can also nurture and support you on this journey.

The process of turning back to yourself can lead to tender and perhaps unfamiliar places within you. As you read the stories of women turning back from self–abandonment, you may recognize your own journey and find yourself feeling open, sensitive, and vulnerable. I recommend reading with your hand on your heart, literally and metaphorically. As you engage with the reflections and exercises that I offer, habits of protection that shielded you in the past may fall away. Be gentle with yourself and support your exploration with love and compassion.

A note of caring caution: If you find that reading this book opens you to overwhelming emotions that are beyond your ability to hold with mindfulness or that require more support than friends and family can offer, I urge you to reach out for professional help. With that guidance you can safely touch the pain of self–abandonment and heal from it.

Although we are each walking our own unique way back to ourselves, we are not walking the path alone. We walk as a community of women who are called back to the fullness of who we are. The path offered in *Turning Back to Ourselves* is imbued with the wisdom of interconnectedness, the understanding that each of our actions affects the people around us and may ripple out into the world in ways that are beyond our comprehension. With that understanding, we walk this path with the intention of being thoughtful and kind in our speech and in our actions, not harming ourselves, our community members, or any other living being.

Healing ourselves is part of healing the world. May our inner transformation and our work in the world foster peace and harmony in our hearts, our homes, and our communities. May it contribute to the end of oppression and the healing of the Earth. The last words of the Buddha to his disciples were "Be a light onto yourself." May *Turning Back to Ourselves* guide you more fully to being that inner light. As you heal, may you open to the sacred mystery of life.

Enjoy the journey—sing, dance, write, be creative, and share your wisdom and joy with the world.

Chapter One

Setting Out on the Journey Back to Ourselves: Understanding Self-Abandonment

Once a year on a Saturday morning in August, several hundred women swim across Cayuga Lake in Upstate New York as a fundraiser for our local hospice. For a number of years, I have participated in this event—playfully and aptly called "Women Swimmin'"—joining with others to support the gentle and compassionate care at the end of life that hospice provides. I am moved by women crossing the lake in memory of their loved ones, their mothers, fathers, life partners, or dear friends. I love seeing the swim caps in all colors of the rainbow bobbing in and out of the water. I am touched by the presence of the boaters in kayaks and canoes who are there to guide and protect us. The swim is deeply personal for me while at the same time connecting me with a community of caring women. This event is one of my favorite days of the year.

But during the first few years I participated in Women Swimmin', I found my excitement tempered by trepidation and self-doubt. I am not a strong athlete, and I would slowly make my way across the 1.2-mile stretch of the lake, continually comparing myself to the other women, telling myself I was not good enough, fearing I might be one of the last to make it to the finish line, questioning whether I should be making this effort at all. *Do I really belong among all these powerful women who seem to be so capable and full of life?* Despite several years of intensive meditation retreats and working off and on with therapists, these ways of thinking about myself, abandoning myself with self-judgment and doubt, were still coming up in my mind. But I eventually arrived at a turning point and the challenging swim across the lake became a way to transform self-abandonment into acceptance and self-love.

In my work now as a therapist and in the women's meditation circle I lead, I see that same pattern of self-judgment and self-doubt coming up over and over. I am struck by how hard it is for women to love themselves and how they turn away from themselves in so many ways and for so many reasons. Remembering my own experience, I listen to their stories with understanding. But I also hear something else from them—something I now know as unshakably true—that no matter how lost we may feel, there is a way to turn back from self-judgment and self-doubt, to remember who we are, and to love ourselves.

We begin our journey back to ourselves by recognizing moments in our lives when we forget we are worthy of love, when we forget we have a place in the world. We begin by noticing times when we lose a sense of connection to ourselves and feel isolated and alienated from everyone and everything. We begin by acknowledging the sense of loss we feel when we are living one step away from ourselves, removed from life. We begin by noticing the fear of presenting ourselves to the world with all our glory ... or all our vulnerabilities. These are moments of self-abandonment. As we recognize them, we also become aware of the pain of being distant from ourselves. We feel the pain of judging, doubting, or hating ourselves. We feel the pain of losing our capacity for joy, peace, and well-being.

In the state of self-abandonment, our emotions might range from mild insecurity to powerful feelings of inadequacy and shame. We might believe that we are inherently flawed, not deserving of love, and that we do not belong anywhere. Women who have abandoned themselves often describe feeling overextended, chronically depressed, or highly anxious. They tell me they feel angry, agitated, or restless, unable to find a peaceful place within themselves. Some feel trapped, believing that the unfulfilling life they are living is the only life they could ever have. Many have little hope for change and are ready to give up on themselves and on their dreams. I hear resignation in their voices and a sense that they are tired of trying.

Kimberly, a nurse at a local hospital, joined my monthly women's circle hoping to find nourishing connections in something outside the usual intensity of her life. Most of the time she arrived at our gatherings exhausted after working her typically long hours each day. She said she had to push herself at home to find the energy to lovingly connect with her partner and her adolescent daughter. "I often feel I have nothing left to give anywhere, but there's this voice inside my head always telling me I should try harder, that I could do more to take better care of my patients and of my family." When I asked her if she ever gives herself some of that same love and support that she gives to others, a pained expression came across her face. "I guess I think that would be selfish," she said.

Anita came to me for counseling because she just couldn't let herself do what she really wanted to do with her life. Passionate about food justice, she had long held a vision of working to promote healthy school lunches for children, and now a local school was seeking a manager for its lunch program. "I have all the right qualifications and I would love the job," Anita said, "but I keep stopping myself from applying—thinking I'd probably not get it ... and who do I think I am anyway?" Despite having been a top student in high school and college, she said she'd never felt smart enough or like she fit in. "Thinking about this job brings up some of those same feelings."

In our first session, Judith told me she hated the way she looked. It started when she was a teenager. "I used to think if only I could get slim, that would be my ticket to acceptance. For a while I did an intense workout routine at home and every Friday night measured my thighs and stomach to make sure I was keeping my weight down." Who she was and whether she could fit in at school seemed to depend entirely on what she recorded each week. But after graduating, that effort broke down, and here she was years later still struggling. "I wish I lived in someone else's body," she said. "In fact, it's everything about me—I don't like who I am."

These women are expressing the pain of so many who have abandoned themselves—whether that has meant caring for others but not themselves, hiding their strengths and talents, or being ashamed of their bodies. Like them, some women have forgotten how to love and cherish themselves; some have never known how. Holding themselves with gentleness and kindness would not occur to them as a response to their pain.

Judging, doubting, or hating ourselves, the hallmarks of self-abandonment, are ways of thinking and feeling that, as the Buddha pointed out, cloud the mind and prevent us from seeing the truth of who we are. When we are caught in self-judgment, it is as if a harsh, scolding voice inside is telling us we are bad, that something is wrong with us, that everything we say or do is not good enough, is unacceptable. Self-doubt is the mindstate that undermines our confidence, dismisses our potential, and questions our sense of belonging—to ourselves, to anyone or anything. It keeps us from expressing ourselves fully and opening to new possibilities. Self-hatred is a painful emotional state that leads us to reject everything about ourselves—our thoughts, our feelings, our right to have a place in the world. For some, like Judith, self-hatred can even manifest as a rejection of their own bodies.

In the presence of these harsh inner voices, there is no space for love, no way we can cherish and rejoice in ourselves, and no way we can freely offer our love to others. We forget what it feels like to be relaxed and at ease in our body and in our mind. We forget there is any other way to be with ourselves or in the world. When we believe these voices, they grow stronger and can lead us into what I call the "downward spiral of self–abandonment." When our negative thoughts continue to feed each other, they take us farther away from loving ourselves. Finding our way out of this downward spiral starts with recognizing the causes that led us to abandon ourselves.

How Did We Get Here?

None of us would choose to turn away from ourselves, but conditions in our lives can lead us there. The causes are often intertwined, layered on top of each other, and it can be difficult to know how to begin unraveling them. As women, some of us abandoned ourselves because that is what we learned from our role models and we didn't know any other way to be. Looking at our mothers and grandmothers, we might have seen women prioritizing the needs of others over their own, sacrificing themselves. They may take on the roles of caretaker, savior, or rescuer, doing more for others than they ever do for themselves. Or we may have heard women around us speaking negatively about themselves, and we have carried those patterns into our own lives. Caught up in any of these habits, we can find ourselves depleted, resentful, bitter, or lacking in joy. Exhausted, we might lash out at the people who are closest to us and then, overcome by guilt and regret, turn against ourselves as well.

Many of us have abandoned ourselves by measuring our behavior and choices against the values and beliefs of those around us. Absorbing their messages about how we should behave, what we should look like, who we should be, we judge ourselves harshly when we fail to meet those expectations, and we lose confidence and trust in our own views and perceptions. We may also abandon ourselves in the face of negative messages about our race, ethnicity, age, abilities, sexual orientation or gender identity. Made to feel "different," we may conclude that we are in some way wrong or incomplete, that we do not belong.

Some of us abandoned ourselves because love and attention were lacking in our homes. According to "attachment theory," developed in the twentieth century by the British psychiatrist and psychotherapist John Bowlby, the way we were treated by our early caregivers affects how as adults we relate to others and, I would add, how we relate to ourselves. If we grew up with what Bowlby calls, "secure attachment," we experienced an environment in which we felt loved and appreciated, our needs were validated and basically met, we developed a basic ease of connection and trust in ourselves and in others. With that foundation, we became open-hearted adults, appreciative, and caring toward ourselves and others. We trust that there is a place for us in the world and that we matter. And as Linda Graham, the author of *Bouncing Back* points out, even though none of us were loved and attuned to at all times, the experience of secure attachment allows us to "bounce back" when we feel hurt or misunderstood, when we encounter the inevitable challenges of life.

But not all of us were raised with the conditions that supported that sense of safety and belonging. Even if our basic needs were met—we had a home to live in, food on the table, clothes to wear, friends to play with—we might not have felt cherished or celebrated. We might not have felt seen or understood. Without that early foundation of support, we would have developed ways to survive and to compensate for what was missing. To get through, some of us closed a part of our heart to ourselves and to the world. Bowlby discerned three attachment styles that arise from the lack of secure attachment.

In some of our families, parents or caregivers were emotionally or physically absent. They may have been preoccupied and distracted, maybe working several jobs to sustain the family, or perhaps caught up in pain, sorrow, or grief. Without receiving adequate love, attention, and caring presence as children, we may have developed a way of relating to others that Bowlby describes as "avoidant" attachment. Concluding that no one would ever be there to care for our needs, we became extremely self-reliant, avoiding reaching out to others for help. As adult women, if we feel that our needs don't matter, we end up feeling that *we ourselves* don't matter.

In other families, love, and care were inconsistent and unreliable. This is what Bowlby calls "ambivalent" or "anxious attachment." Not understanding why our parents or caregivers were warm and loving one day and completely unavailable the next, we might have blamed ourselves. *There must be something wrong with me if they loved me yesterday but don't love me today.* Losing confidence and trust in ourselves, our sense of self-worth became dependent on the praise or the approval of others. As adult women, in order to avoid conflict with others or feelings of abandonment, we might apologize profusely and feel compelled to please and appease others. Some women who have had this kind of upbringing say they feel a constant hollow space in their heart that longs to be filled.

And some of us grew up in homes where there were actual threats to our body and to the core sense of who we are. We might have been abused and shamed by the very people we expected to be loved and protected by. Or we might have grown up in constant fear of an eruption of anger or violence. Some of us were sexually assaulted. In response, we developed what Bowlby called "disorganized attachment." We may have spent much of our childhood just trying to survive, trying to find ways to cope, to shelter, to defend ourselves from harm, and to understand a world that did not make sense to us. We might have tried to survive by fighting back or running away. Or we silenced ourselves, made ourselves small so as not to provoke more harm. Some of us dissociated, disconnecting from our bodies and hearts, so we would not feel the horror of mistreatment or abuse. As adult women, we might still be emotionally guarded, not daring to expose our vulnerability. We might find ourselves in tumultuous relationships, reenacting some of what we experienced in childhood. We may get lost in emotional reactivity or completely shut down our feelings.

Any of these environments in our childhood could have left us abandoning ourselves, not fulfilling our potential or our dreams. For some of us these experiences were traumatizing and may still be having an impact on our lives as adults. Peter Levine, a leading trauma therapist and author of *Waking the Tiger*, defines trauma as "something that overwhelms us, that makes us feel helpless, that makes us feel paralyzed. And it's something that happens to our bodies and our brains, something that happens to our nervous system, to our whole organism, that doesn't un–happen."

Women who have suffered severe trauma often speak of losing their zest for life and disconnecting from their potential for joy and vitality. Many never feel safe in their body, always scanning for danger. Others suffer from high levels of anxiety and depression. Some have a strong need to control their environment as a way of protecting themselves. Some turn to self–harming behaviors, such as cutting, burning, starving themselves, overeating, or other forms of addiction to numb their feelings. When traumatic events of this kind are not healed, these women may lose their sense of wholeness, as if a part of themselves has been left behind.

Levine points out that there are milder forms of trauma that often get overlooked as small and insignificant events, something that 'just happens to all of us," something we need to "just get over," such as being mocked by a friend in the schoolyard, losing a pet, our parents yelling at us in anger, or the sense of being different and not belonging. But while these milder forms of trauma don't necessarily hold us back from successfully engaging in our lives, they may show up as those voices in our minds that doubt or judge us. They may give rise to spikes of anxiety or anger, or numbness. They may erode our confidence and turn us away from loving ourselves.

Any unresolved trauma, whether it is minor or severe, can lead to self–abandonment. And if traumatic events happened repeatedly, especially during our childhood when we may have lacked protection and support, they can have an even more powerful impact on who we are now as women. In response to that trauma, we may turn away from the parts of ourselves that are hurting, lose touch with our needs, our dreams, our aliveness, and our joy. Shut down spiritually and emotionally, we may hide our vibrant inherent creativity under layers of fear, anger, guilt, or shame and grow distant from ourselves, from others, and from life. As we feel the pain of self-abandonment and meet it with an open heart, compassion arises in us and, from that tender place, we begin our turn back. We turn back from the habit of judging ourselves as bad or wrong, from doubting and rejecting ourselves. We turn back from living with limitations and fear and take ourselves back into our hearts. No matter how many times we have lost our way or how far we have gone in the wrong direction, we can always turn back. We can turn back toward home.

While our personal history and the messages we have received about what it means to be a woman may have led us to self-abandonment, held us back from manifesting our innate beauty, and kept us from loving and trusting ourselves, each of our stories has brought us to this point where we begin our journey back to ourselves. For any of us lost in the downward spiral, there comes a moment when we recognize that there is indeed a way out. This moment might arise as a sudden insight when we see clearly how we are limiting ourselves and we choose to no longer do so. It can come when the pain we are experiencing is too much to bear and we reach out for help. This awakening may dawn on us when we are in nature or when we are touched by a dear friend who brings us back to who we are. It might happen in a burst of creativity or in a moment when we experience a profound connection to life around us. Even if we catch a glimpse of what it feels like to take ourselves back into our hearts but then lose track of it, we know we have seen the possibility of finding our way back.

The Wise and Compassionate Self

At some point, in the midst of our dissatisfaction, we hear the calling to turn back to ourselves. Some of us are called back by a yearning for love, for inner peace, for happiness and aliveness, or by a desire to know how we can make a positive difference in the world. Some of us are called back to ourselves because we are hurting, suffering physically or emotionally, because something in our lives is not working. Some of us are called by a thirst for the truth, a wish to find answers to existential questions about life and death, questions about time and space, questions about the nature of the mind, or by a longing for the sacred. Whatever the reason for this call, it is the part of ourselves that remembers our innate goodness and knows we are worthy of love that is inviting us to return. I call her the "wise and compassionate self."

In Buddhist teachings, the qualities of wisdom and compassion are sometimes referred to as the two wings of a bird, both needed and working together so that the bird can fly. Wisdom sees clearly the nature of life, recognizing that all experiences inside and around us are constantly changing and that freedom and happiness arise from letting go of wanting things to be a certain way. Compassion is the quality of heart that opens us to feel our pain and the pain of others and motivates us to take action to alleviate that suffering.

Living in touch with our wise and compassionate self opens us to holding ourselves and all of life with love. We may feel her presence as a gentle vibration in our chest or a fullness of heart. We may know her as the warmth of love, the relaxation of self–acceptance, or the grounded feeling of belonging. We may experience her as quietude, inner peace, calm, ease, and contentment. In her presence our hearts are filled with kindness, gratitude, creativity, and joy. She is the presence within us that leads us out of self–abandonment.

As we turn back to ourselves, we open to her presence in our lives. When we meet her and get to know her, some of the old habits of distancing from ourselves are transformed. Instead of judging and doubting ourselves, we hold ourselves tenderly with an open heart. Instead of dismissing and ignoring our needs, we listen and care for ourselves.

We might imagine this part of us as a lighthearted joyful woman singing and dancing, fully present, fully alive. We might imagine her as the elder wise woman of the village or the kind matriarch of the family. She is centered, clear, and warm. She is the part of ourselves in which we can take refuge, the part of ourselves with whom we feel protected, cared for, and safe. She listens carefully to our thoughts, feelings, and needs, and in her wisdom, she guides us toward happiness. She is forgiving of mistakes, always ready to stand by our side as an ally or a friend, as we learn and start again. She is the one we rediscover each time we turn back from self-abandonment. She is wisdom deeper than thinking, and her compassion is boundless in soothing the pain of the heart.

This part of ourselves has been recognized in many spiritual and healing traditions as the embodiment of the essence of who we are. She has been called the centered self, the core self, the highest self, the authentic or the true self. Some speak of her as a spark of God within us. No matter what name we may use, touching into this essence is our lived experience of connection to the sacred.

In my therapy practice and women's circles, I ask them how they experience this part of themselves. Some, feeling overwhelmed by the difficulties in their lives, may begin by saying they have no access to a part of themselves that feels the kind of love and connection I'm talking about. But when we explore the question a little longer, most begin to recall a time when they felt at home within themselves, a time when they felt at ease and connected to life. Many say they long for that part of themselves but don't know how to find her.

There are some women who do readily recall a moment when they knew their wise and compassionate self. They describe feeling alive, in the flow, free of obstruction and confinement. They speak of feeling light and tall, big versus small, present instead of distracted. They talk about feeling a life force moving through them and being able to express themselves fully and freely. Some speak of experiencing an expanded sense of time, or timelessness. Others relate a vast sense of self that includes mountains, rivers, oceans, the sky, and all living beings. In recounting these moments of touching into the wise and compassionate self, they say things like: "I had arrived" or "Everything had fallen into place."

Remembering our wise and compassionate self can happen at any moment, right in the middle of our lives. We might be diving under a wave, sitting on our porch listening to the birds, or walking down a busy city street. We discover her in solitude, and we may know her in relationships with others. In her presence, for a moment we let go of striving for some image of ourselves. We simply surrender to who we are.

> ### Remembering Your Wise and Compassionate Self
>
> Let yourself call to mind a time when you felt love flowing through you, a time when you felt connected to a sense of something greater than yourself. You might have been walking in nature, deep in meditation, working in your garden, or teaching a class. What did you feel in your body? What was the state of your mind? As you touch into this experience of your wise and compassionate self, ask what message she might have for you now. Notice what her response awakens in you, and then carry that feeling with you as you return to your day.

Abiding in our wise and compassionate selves does not mean that we deny suffering and challenges in our lives and consider only pleasant experiences as acceptable. That would be denying the truth of our human existence. When we are in physical or emotional pain, instead of distancing from ourselves, we can reach out to this part of ourselves and meet those difficult experiences with kindness, courage, understanding, and love.

No matter how near or far our wise and compassionate self may seem at any given moment, we can trust that she is always there, present as a deep and true part of ourselves. Even if she is concealed or forgotten for a period of time, we can always find our way back to her again.

Life Give Us Clues

Recently looking through a box of memorabilia, I came upon a photograph of myself at about two years old, held in my mother's arms. I look comfortable and secure, my face radiating ease, trust, and aliveness. Clearly, I was in the paradise of innocence where the world was whole, and I was part of it. Held by what psychologist Bill Plotkin refers to as "uncompromised love," I was protected and safe, abiding in a sense of unity and oneness with the world. Held in the loving arms of my family, I carried that sense of security into my early adventures. So even when my family moved from South Africa to Israel when I was five years old, I was eager and ready to explore. Within six months, I was speaking Hebrew and joining other children running along the paths and playing in the fields on the edge of the village where we lived. I had an unquestioned sense of belonging.

But when I was about to turn eight years old, my family moved again to a new town. The resilience I had learned in my home would find its first real challenge in this new and unfamiliar world. My first day there, I walked down the stairs of our new apartment building, expecting to find someone to play with, but my attempt to connect with the next-door neighbor girl who was about my age did not bear fruit. Disappointed but still hopeful, a few days later I started school, expecting to make friends, to be loved, to be happy. The other children had known each other since they were infants, and they didn't need a new friend. I felt confused, lonely, and out of place. I experienced a puzzling dissonance between the deep love and acceptance I knew at home and the sense of separation and alienation I felt at school. For the first time, I began to question: *Do I fit in? Where do I belong?* That was my first taste of what self-abandonment means. I began doubting myself, trying to please others and seek their approval. I began to lose touch with my sense of wholeness and belonging, and I did not know how to get it back.

The question of belonging followed me through my adolescence. There were moments of feeling part of a group and other times when I felt out of place, not connected to the people I was with. One evening sitting around the table with my friends at a field study center where I lived and worked for a couple of years, someone mentioned one of the young men who worked with us. "I love him," I said innocently—and there was a loud burst of laughter. What had I said wrong? In my home we often freely expressed love for people we cared about. I felt confused and hurt. My chest tightened and tears began stinging my eyes. Did I really belong in this group? And if I didn't belong here either, then who was I and where did I fit in?

Many of us might remember a time in our childhood when we stepped out of the protection of our family into the wider world. For the first time we may have experienced ourselves as a "separate" self, no longer feeling part of a larger whole. Or we might recall those times in our adolescence when we felt self-conscious, concerned about what others thought of us, and out of touch with any positive ways we regarded ourselves.

This loss of the sense of wholeness, the seed of self-abandonment, can also at the same time be the place where our healing journey begins. Diana Fosha, trauma therapist, author, and creator of Accelerated Experiential Dynamic Psychotherapy (AEDP), says that despite the challenges we encounter in our lives, we all have within us an "innate motivational drive to heal, self-right, and flourish." The image she offers to represent this is a flower finding its way to the sun through cracks in the sidewalk. It is this innate force that Fosha calls "transformation" that puts us on the path back to ourselves.

We may not know quite what we are looking for or how to solve the restlessness inside, but life keeps providing us with clues, though we may only notice them when we are ready. We might walk into a bookstore and "accidentally" find the book that will pique our curiosity and get us interested in a path back to ourselves. We might see a sign on our college campus for a talk that will open the door to a new life. We might hear a song that touches a chord in our heart and gives us the courage to take the step we know we must. When we are ready, the clues fall into our hands, like plucking ripe berries off a bush.

A memorable moment that set me on the path back to myself happened in my late teens with the visit of one of my mother's hippie cousins. Each summer in Israel our young adult relatives would arrive with their backpacks and guitars and sleep on mattresses on our front porch. I was fascinated by their stories of distant lands. One cousin, Daryl, was in his twenties, and I was interested in everything he had to say. When he told us he'd been practicing something called "meditation," I was intrigued. He seemed happy and calm. "It's hard to describe," he said in response to my questions. "It's like salt. You don't know what it tastes like until you've tried it." I had no idea what he meant, but the thought of sitting still and turning inward called to something deep within me.

Shortly after, I came across a book about Buddhism. It was difficult to read, but I stuck with it. As I finished the last pages, I found myself sobbing. I remember walking my dog Jerry through the streets of our neighborhood, tears streaming down my face. I did not know why I was crying. I only knew my heart was touched, and I wanted to know more about this thing people were hinting at. I wanted to know how I could find it for myself.

I certainly had experienced a taste of this "something" at moments in my life—lighting the candles on Friday night and singing "Kiddush" to welcome in Shabbat was one of them. Those moments with my family always opened the door to the experience of something I recognized as sacred. And in moments of walking in the desert at the end of a day of hiking, the golden light of the setting sun reflecting off the hills, my heart would be touched by beauty and a sense of something larger than myself. But despite such beautiful moments, underneath was that persistent feeling of not fitting in, not being sure where I belonged. I was longing for what could help me find my way back to what I knew must be there. The stories Daryl was telling about meditation practice seemed to be offering a clue about what could lead me there.

Then one day a friend told me that his sister Roni had just come back from India. "I think you'll find she has some understanding about what you're looking for," he said. I took a bus to the kibbutz where Roni lived in the north of Israel, and we spent an afternoon talking on a shady porch, covered by a canopy of grapevines. The sound of wind blowing through the vines added to the feeling of serenity as she shared her stories with me. We spread out a map of India and Nepal on the wicker table, and she showered me with travel tips. Then, toward the end of the afternoon, she told me the story I knew I had come for.

During her travels, Roni had participated in a ten-day silent retreat in Bodh Gaya, the place where the Buddha is said to have attained enlightenment. She described the small village that hosted Buddhist monasteries from many countries around the world including and the Thai monastery where the retreat took place. She told me about the schedule, sitting and walking in silence, cultivating moment-to-moment awareness throughout the day. I was touched by the trust she conveyed in the teachers and the teaching, and her confidence in the path she had found. More than the details of the retreat, what I took away from that conversation was the sense of inner stillness and calm that Roni radiated.

This was the signpost I had been waiting for. A strong intention welled up in me to venture out and explore for myself the path to peace and happiness that Roni had described. I had been wandering in a maze of self-abandonment for a long time, and now I could see the way out. I was going to India and Nepal to discover that path, that deeper understanding of life that was calling to me. I would find the path back to myself.

Finding a path back to ourselves is part of our journey. It might take time, some inquiry and discernment to find the one that inspires us and that we choose to follow. But when we come across the way that calls us, we set out on a quest for our authentic self. This journey invariably takes us beyond the boundaries of the known and the familiar. For some it is a physical journey in which we leave behind the comfort of our home, our family, and our friends and venture to new lands. For others it is a journey of the mind and the heart departing from old habits of thinking and being. Setting off on this journey back to ourselves requires courage and faith, the willingness to step into the unknown to look for something we might not even know we are seeking. It is the beginning of turning back to ourselves.

Setting a Wise Intention

Turning back to our wise and compassionate self begins when we recognize that we must do something to change our life, to end the pain of turning against ourselves. Despite whatever difficulty we are facing, we recognize the preciousness of our life and the possibility of living in a different way. It is as if our wise and compassionate self is knocking on the doors of our heart urging us to wake up. In those moments an intention arises in us to turn back to ourselves with kindness and love, to find our way back home.

Setting an intention means consciously choosing the direction we are headed in our life. It is like standing on the deck of a ship, holding a compass in one hand and the steering wheel in the other, now heading steadily in the direction of home. Our intention is our North Star, guiding us even when the winds and the currents are strong and want to pull us off course. Knowing at last where we are going, we remain focused, clear, and purposeful.

The intention to turn back to ourselves is based in the faith that we can and will find our way back. We begin to clarify not only what we want to leave behind but also what we are yearning for. We find the words that express not only the direction we're going but also how we intend to get there. We may set an intention to hold ourselves with love, to speak to ourselves kindly, and to no longer judge ourselves. We may set an intention to care for our body and our mind. Or we may set an intention to do no harm to others and to not be silent in the face of injustice. We set our intention in words that can remind us to turn back when old habits arise and we forget that we have chosen to embark on a new path back to ourselves.

Setting an intention doesn't necessarily mean that we can control how our journey unfolds or demand that life proceeds in the way we want it to. There will be times when we are thrown off course by thoughts and feelings of self-abandonment, but with the support of our intention, we realign ourselves with our direction back to our wise and compassionate self.

When our intention is clear, whenever we feel we have lost our way, we can pause and ask ourselves: *Am I going in the right direction? Is this action that I am about to perform aligned with my intention? Is this action imbued with love? Will it support me in turning back to myself, or will it deepen the habits of self-abandonment?* Asking ourselves these questions helps us realign with our intention and sets us back on course.

The intention to turn back from self-abandonment, to not give up on ourselves, is revolutionary. It is a bold step away from feeling that we don't matter. It is a statement of valuing and honoring ourselves, a declaration of trust in ourselves, a commitment to ourselves, and a willingness to face whatever inner demons are trying to persuade us otherwise. With kindness we choose to turn back to ourselves, remembering our innate worth and beauty, remembering our commitment to grow in wisdom and understanding and to live a life of non-harming. Setting an intention to turn back to ourselves motivates us, energizes us, and gives us the courage to move forward.

Setting the Intention to Turn Back to Your Wise and Compassionate Self

In this reflection you will be discovering how you might want to state your intention to turn back to yourself. Having pen and paper to write that down would be most helpful. Begin with a few moments to settle in, taking a few deep and easy breaths. Then bring your attention to your heart center and ask yourself: *What is the calling of my heart?* You might be yearning for love, peace, understanding, creative expression. Let the words arise that express the longings of your heart. Your words may be *I set the intention to open my heart to myself… to live with kindness … to hold my pain with compassion.* When you have found the intentions that feel right, repeat them to yourself several times, either silently or aloud. Notice what you feel in your body and in your heart as you say these words. It can be most helpful to repeat your phrases when you wake up in the morning and before you go to sleep. Notice throughout your day how setting your intention affects your actions and opens your heart.

Setting an intention can also be likened to sowing a seed in our garden. It is not enough to just put the seed in the ground and leave it there. We need to tend it, water and nourish the soil, then protect the new seedling and support it as it grows. Each time we recite our intention, we are nurturing the seeds of the kindness and care we wish to cultivate. Bringing the seeds of intention to fruition requires careful ongoing attention. There are many paths and practices that can support us in this process. You might be drawn to yoga, qigong, or tai chi as you support your intention to nurture your body. Meditation, the contemplative practices of some religions, or shamanic and pagan healing practices might offer a foundation and pathway for your heart and spirit. Being in nature, gardening, or playing music might be the path that leads you back to yourself. Whatever calls you, dedicating yourself with intention is what will take you home to your wise and compassionate self.

Realigning with Our Intention

One year our family arrived back in New York after a long transatlantic flight from Israel. It was very early morning and still dark when we left the airport to drive home to Ithaca, 250 miles upstate. Longing to get home, we merged onto the freeway heading north. Ian was driving, and I was in the back seat with our two daughters, Tamar and Noa, both curled up around me sleeping. Somewhere along the way we pulled into a rest stop for a few minutes. Then, jet lagged and somewhat fuzzy minded, we got back on the road. I was struggling to stay awake, staring ahead at the road stretching out before us. At some point I noticed that Ian was trying to catch my eye in the rearview mirror, pointing backward with his thumb. Puzzled but not wanting to disturb the girls by talking, I just waited and watched as he took the next exit, slowed down, turned left onto the overpass, and then merged back onto the freeway heading the opposite way. The message was clear. Since the rest stop, we'd been going in the wrong direction for miles and miles. Course correction needed. The only way to get us home was a U-turn.

We all have those signs in our lives that wake us up and tell us we are going the wrong direction, abandoning ourselves again. These might be waves of high anxiety, racing thoughts, overwhelming depression, arguments with our family members, a sudden episode of road rage, or feelings of deep discomfort in our bodies. These feelings wake us up and tell us that it is time to slow down and turn around. They remind us of what we already know—that the habits of self-abandonment will not lead us to happiness. The direction we are going will not take us home to ourselves, will not lead us to inner peace but only take us farther and farther away from where we are longing to be. And so, holding ourselves with love and compassion, we awaken and turn back to ourselves.

The journey we undertake is not to a faraway land but, rather, to the truth of who we are. On this journey we turn and take ourselves back into our hearts. Kimberly would discover what it meant to lovingly care for herself. Anita would find the trust in herself to take on the position she wanted as manager of the school-lunch program. And as Judith slowly transformed her feelings about her body, she joined a sports club and discovered that she actually enjoyed being physically active. As we begin to turn back to ourselves, we enter the upward spiral that brings us back to our true and vibrant selves.

Women Swimmin' was my upward spiral. As I prepared for the fourth year of my participation in the fundraiser, I chose a new way of relating to myself and to my habitual defeating thoughts. During the weeks before the event, each time I went down to the lake to practice swimming, I also practiced "turning back to myself." As I slathered my arms and legs with olive oil to keep warm in the early June waters, I practiced remaining aware of that inner voice of self-doubt that tried to hold me back. *I should be home taking care of the family and the house. I'm not a good swimmer—Why am I even trying? Maybe I should just not do the swim this year.* No matter what that voice was saying, I kept reminding myself that this experience was a way to turn back to myself with love. And in those moments, love meant getting in the water and swimming.

One evening a week before the event, I made my way to the water with a strong intention to honor my efforts and my ability without judgment, to love myself for showing up yet again. Instead of getting caught in negative self-judgment, I turned my attention to the moment. As I waded in, I noticed the smooth feeling of water on my skin and noticed the little bubbles of air forming in the olive oil barrier on my legs. After standing up to my knees in the cold water for a few minutes, I jumped in. What a thrill! A gentle vibration rippled down my spine. I paused for a moment to catch my breath and to appreciate the courage it took to turn away from doubting myself and just dive in.

For the first few minutes of swimming, my mind kept slipping into self-judgment—*I haven't accomplished enough today, I said the wrong thing to that person, I'm such a slow swimmer.* Each time I noticed those thoughts, I shifted my attention back to the sensations in my body, feeling the movement of my arms and legs and the rhythm of my breathing. In those moments of being present, of not letting myself get caught in undermining thoughts, I was turning back to myself. This was a triumph as meaningful as accomplishing the swim across the lake would be.

During the rest of that week leading up to the event, each time I arrived at the lake, my heart was filled with joy. The sunsets were breathtaking, the orange–pink sky reflecting in the water like a painting in a museum. My heart opened with gratitude for the beauty and for being alive. I trusted my ability to cross the lake without judging myself as wrong or out of place. I was ready in my own way now to make the long swim with the other women, to contribute my strength and vitality to the beautiful cause of the event … and this time I would do it without turning against myself.

The day of the swim arrived. My eyes were teary as I walked down the steep road to the lakeshore, greeted along the way by those who were there to support and cheer on the swimmers. I took in the warmth and kindness they radiated, feeling held and cared for. As we heard the signal to begin, we all entered the water and started making our way across the lake. This year, for the first time, I was not constantly comparing myself to the other swimmers or judging myself as good or bad. When I got tired in the middle of the lake, rather than berating myself, I slowed down, turned to float on my back, looked around, and rested a little. I took in the beautiful panorama of distant hills surrounding the lake and the vast expansive space around me. A few times the thought *She is swimming faster than me* briefly crossed my mind, but for once it did not take center stage. Feeling my body slowly moving through the water, I commended myself with a smile: *I can only swim the breaststroke, but nonetheless, I am swimming!"*

When I approached the ladder to climb back up to the dock, my family was waiting for me. I could not stop my tears as my body trembled gently from the effort and excitement. I felt happy, relieved, and accomplished. Looking around me, meeting the eyes of other swimmers, I saw joy, warmth, and vulnerability. I saw women being visible, strong, and capable, and I was one of them. Seeing women so deeply connected to themselves and being kind and supportive of each other during that event reminded me of what I know is possible for women when we choose to turn back to ourselves. I felt the power of transformation that arises when we hold ourselves with kindness, compassion, and love. Standing by the water wrapped in a towel, looking back across the distance I had managed to cross, I was filled with gratitude.

Habits of self-abandonment might not let go easily. We might need to turn back to ourselves again and again with courage, perseverance, and patience, but eventually the scales tip, and even when we experience difficult mindstates, we no longer abandon ourselves. We turn back and reclaim our wise and compassionate self. As we let love, compassion, joy, and wisdom effortlessly flow through us, we know a deep sense of connection to ourselves and to the world around us. When our heart is open in this way, we remember that we are worthy of love. We know from within that we are connected to ourselves and to each other, and we know we are always welcome on this Earth.

CHAPTER TWO

Bringing Our Attention to the Present: Turning Back with Mindfulness

Inspired by my conversation with Roni, I began preparations for India. Ready to welcome a new "me," I had my hair cut short. I put only the bare minimum into my backpack—a few T-shirts, light skirts, sandals, my favorite water bottle, and a journal. I said my goodbyes to my family at a cookout on one of our favorite beaches. The feeling of the sand between my toes and the salty sea breeze were a reminder of the many evenings of my childhood when I'd played in the waves, watching the golden sun disappear on the horizon. I would now be entering a new phase of my life. While I sensed a slight nervousness in those who had come to wish me well, inwardly I felt confident, excited, and imbued with the thrill of adventure.

First, the mountains of Nepal called me. I joined some friends to climb up to Gokyo Peak, a 17,575-foot-high mountain southwest of Mount Everest. We started our trek in the foothills of the Himalayas and followed narrow paths through misty forests and small picturesque villages. Then I took a detour and made my way on my own to Tengboche, a Tibetan Buddhist monastery. After spending the night in a tiny guest room, I was awakened by the deep sound of the long brass horns that call the monks to their daily rituals. The vibration echoed through me, drawing me inward, toward something I deeply longed for.

As I continued toward Gokyo Peak, the climb grew more intense. In the high altitude, breathing was labored, and each step required effort. I walked slowly, placing one foot in front of the other, the strenuous climb forcing me to pay attention to each breath and each step. Being present in this way seemed to bring me closer to myself and to a sense of what I was seeking.

The view from the top of the mountain was vast and expansive, white waves of snow extending as far as I could see. Black ravens glided on air currents below us. Sitting in silence, my heart opened and I was filled with awe. With a sense of promise and possibility, I started the long walk back down the mountain. I was now ready to do what I came to Asia for, to find an answer to the longing of my heart.

I arrived at the village of Bodh Gaya after dark on a chilly December night. The rickshaw driver dropped me off at the Burmese Vihara, the pilgrimage hostel that opened its doors to Western travelers. It would be a few days until the next retreat would begin, so I had time to explore the village. I made friends with other young people, and we spent our days talking about our journeys. In the early evenings as the sun was setting, we would make our way to the Japanese Zen temple. As we sat cross–legged facing a statue of the Buddha, monks in long black robes walked around the room, correcting our posture and from time to time yelling out words I could not understand. The physical pain of the sitting posture invariably grew more intense during the forty–five minutes of stillness, but at the end of the meditation, my whole body would reverberate with the sound of the gong. My mind would be calm and my heart lighter.

After dinner I would join the Tibetan pilgrims in their practice of walking around the Mahabodhi Temple, the Temple of Great Awakening, built on the site of the Buddha's enlightenment. My heart was moved by the commitment and devotion of these practitioners as they turned prayer wheels, reciting mantras to cultivate compassion. Walking silently with them, the darkness lit by flickering oil lamps in small niches in the walls of the compound, I felt touched by the sacred. I was walking in the footsteps of thousands of seekers who had come here before me looking for the same relief from suffering.

Then the day I was waiting for arrived. I stepped into the Thai temple to take part in a meditation retreat. The conversation I'd had with Daryl when I was a teenager, meeting Roni, and the heart opening I felt sitting at the top of Gokyo Peak looking out into the open expanse— all had guided me to this moment and this place. I was joining eighty travelers from around the world who had come together, all led by the same calling, to deepen our understanding and to open our hearts to true happiness. Some, like me, were new to meditation, others were experienced dharma students, but we were all there with the same intention. During that afternoon, we entered the meditation hall and carefully placed our pillows and blankets on the floor, each of us setting up the spot that would be our "home" for the next ten days. When the bell rang that evening to mark the beginning of the retreat, we settled into our places, ready, as we'd been instructed, to keep our eyes to ourselves and talk to no one but the teachers and, if necessary, the staff, in order to immerse ourselves in our own practice.

As the rustle and sounds of everyone adjusting their shawls and meditation postures slowly subsided, we entered what felt like a sacred silence. Here it was, the moment I had been waiting for. I was filled with excitement, and anticipation. We were warmly welcomed by the teacher, Christopher Titmuss. I felt a little thrill in my heart each time I heard him refer to "the path" or "the truth." I had arrived, now part of the *sangha*, the community of like-minded people all seeking what I had been searching for.

Christopher gave us the first instructions in the practice of mindfulness —*vipassana* in the language of the Buddha, meaning insight or seeing clearly. He explained that this was the oldest of the Buddhist meditation practices, originating in India 2,600 years ago. Something about this ancient practice called to me. I was open and ready to learn.

What Is Mindfulness?

In Buddhist teachings, mindfulness is described as a faculty of mind that observes and knows what we are experiencing in the moment, holding it with a spacious, nonreactive awareness. With mindfulness we are aware of the whole array of our inner and outer experiences without shying away from nor clinging to any of them. Mindful awareness has been compared to a mirror that reflects back what it sees. No matter what is put in front of the mirror, the mirror itself remains clear, not taking on the images it is reflecting. In the same way, mindfulness sees what is arising but is not changed or affected by any of it, nor does it change or affect what it sees. Like a mirror, mindfulness does not have an agenda and does not have preferences. It simply notices what is before it.

Mindfulness practice is one of the main tools we use to turn back to ourselves. When we direct our attention to whatever our experience is in the moment, we are reversing the habit of turning away from ourselves. With mindfulness we listen to our inner experience, honoring and respecting ourselves, accepting and allowing ourselves to be just who we are even when we are lost in painful thoughts and emotions. I have come to think of mindfulness as a loving awareness that is clear and nonreactive while at the same time warm, caring, and embracing. When we turn toward our experience and meet it with this awareness, compassion for ourselves arises and we can hold our pain with kindness and care.

Mindfulness is an intentional relationship we have with ourselves and with our experience. In this relationship we choose to turn back to ourselves moment by moment and meet our experience with open eyes and an open heart. We choose to rest our attention on sensations in our body, on our thoughts and feelings. We choose to hold our experience with loving awareness, without judgment.

Mindfulness protects us from falling into habits of self–abandonment. When we are mindful, we readily see ways we are distancing from ourselves or treating ourselves unkindly. We might notice those inclinations as tension in our bodies and in our minds. We might become aware of them as judgments and thoughts that undermine us. We might notice that we are lost in strong waves of fear or anger, numbness or indifference. When we observe these mindstates of self–abandonment with awareness, not feeding them or adding to them, not believing them, we find that they begin to dissipate and lose their power over us. As we shine the light of awareness on thoughts and emotions arising from self–abandonment, we see that they are not permanent and they are not who we truly are. We learn that we do not need to fear them, nor do we need to hold onto them.

Mindfulness helps us see which of our thoughts, emotions, and behaviors lead to self–abandonment and which lead us back to our wise and compassionate selves. With that clarity we are able to choose which qualities of mind and heart we wish to cultivate and which to let go of. We can choose kindness over harshness, self–acceptance over self–judgment, love and compassion over hatred and rejection. As we make those wise choices moment by moment, we turn back to ourselves.

With mindfulness we learn to reconnect with ourselves right in the midst of our lives and to free ourselves from the tangles of negative emotions and hurtful stories. With practice, mindfulness becomes our way of being in the world. We are no longer going through our days in a haze, but awake and aware, we are present and able to respond to ourselves and to all forms of life with kindness, compassion, and care. This is what I would begin to learn on that mindfulness retreat in India.

Paying Attention Moment by Moment

That first evening I listened carefully, eagerly taking in what Christopher was teaching. We were invited to pay attention to our actual experience, noticing what was happening moment by moment. We were encouraged to carry a thread of mindfulness throughout each of the ten days of the retreat, from the time we woke up in the morning until we lay down to sleep at night. We were guided to keep being mindful during sitting and walking meditation, during breaks, and during meals. The instruction was to be present with one thing at a time: just breathing, just hearing, just tasting. Just being. I listened carefully. The teaching and the meditation instructions were promising that being mindful would lead to peace, happiness, and well-being. I listened with a smile on my face, taking it all in. This is what I had come for.

But I soon learned that turning inward with mindfulness on this journey of self-discovery would require more than eagerness and curiosity. It would take courage to continue turning my attention inward and getting to know the inner landscape of my thoughts and feelings. It would take honesty to see myself clearly and not hide behind an image I wanted to uphold. And it would take perseverance to continue walking this sometimes-challenging path and to trust that the practice of mindfulness would lead me to what my heart longed for.

My intention to find that path had led me here, but it was only as I started paying attention to my mind that I knew why I had actually come. I had heard the Buddha's teaching about suffering and the causes of suffering, but now I would begin to realize what that really meant. I would experience the agitation of the wanting mind, the restlessness of the frustrated mind, and the confusion of the deluded mind. And I would experience a pain I knew well but had not been able to give a name to—not being at home within myself.

In the silence, it would be me and my mind, me and my thoughts, me and my heart. There was nowhere to hide. I would have to admit to myself that I was not accustomed to being present with myself in this way. I would have to keep reminding myself that I was taking my first steps on a new path. I would have to practice being patient and giving myself room to grow.

The following morning the bell rang at 5:00 a.m. and we began our first full day of meditation. We were asked to pay attention to the sensations of the movement of our breath, to notice the expansion of our abdomen and chest with the in-breath and the contraction with the out-breath, to notice when the breath was deep and smooth and when it felt shallow and tight. I practiced diligently, but I began noticing that each time I brought my attention to the movement of the breath, within seconds my mind would be off thinking about something entirely unrelated. I'd return my attention back to the breath, and again it would slip away. The same thing happened when we began practicing walking meditation, slowly placing each step with careful attention. *Lifting, moving, placing.* Over and over I had to bring my attention back to the sensations of each step.

Over the next days of the retreat, the meditation instructions continued to expand our field of awareness. We opened to our senses, noticing sounds, sights, smells, tastes, textures. During walking meditation, which we practiced outdoors, I discovered beauty where I had not seen it before. I noticed the light of the sun reflecting off the golden roof of the temple. I listened to the sound of birds in the early morning. I heard the vendors calling out their merchandise, selling bananas, peanuts, and Indian sweets. Their voices and the rattle of their carts rolling down the road felt like background music accompanying the silence of the retreat. I felt the softness of the Nepali wool shawl I was wrapped in, enjoying the texture of the fabric as it touched my skin. At mealtimes, the smells and tastes of the delicious food were a special delight. I looked forward to those meals, a daily highlight of the retreat. And I had glimmers of the joy of being awake and aware, the joy of knowing things as they are, being present with my actual experience in the moment.

Then we were invited to explore sensations throughout our bodies and to simply notice that some were pleasant, some were unpleasant, and some were neutral. The movement of my breath was not especially pleasant nor unpleasant, but other sensations clearly were feelings I either wanted more of or wanted to avoid. I struggled with tightness in my back and the unpleasant tingling when my foot would fall asleep from sitting still for so long with my legs crossed. I was intrigued by the subtle vibrations I felt in my head and the waves of energy that sometimes seemed to be pushing my body over. I was discovering a whole world I had not noticed before: pleasant tingling or warmth moving down my arms or back, heaviness in my chest, pressure in my stomach, tightness in my throat. As I paid close attention to those sensations, I saw that they were not static—they were alive, vibrating, pulsating, rising and falling away, moment by moment. I felt like I was reclaiming my body.

Listening to the talks, I felt the teachers were speaking directly to me. These ancient teachings felt as relevant now as they must have been to the disciples sitting at the feet of the Buddha. I saw in myself the suffering he talked about and recognized the causes he revealed, and I was learning to walk the path he offered to relieve that suffering. I was inspired by my teachers who had been walking this path for many years. They were kind and wise, and in their very being they were showing me where the path could lead to. Even though I didn't yet understand much about what they meant by "inner freedom," there were moments when I began to get a taste of a calmer mind and a sense of the peace and understanding being offered by the teachings.

In the next step after attending to sensations in the body, we were asked to expand our field of awareness and pay attention to mindstates. Just as with other objects of attention, we were to be mindful of them arising and passing away, without clinging to them or resisting. I learned to recognize the brightness of the mind when I was well rested, and the foggy, dreamy mind when tired. There were moments of my mind feeling settled and calm while watching my breath or walking on the grounds, and other times when my mind was restless, unable to be present. There were moments of clarity when I could hear the teachings and understand them, and other moments of confusion when the teachings felt abstract and ungraspable. I noticed how those mindstates appeared and disappeared, constantly changing.

Then we learned how to recognize emotions and the way they manifest in the body. I noticed an expansion in my chest when I was filled with joy, or my heart swelling with gratitude for the generosity of the cooks and the managers of the retreat, or the rush of excitement when I would catch sight of Vincent, a man I had just met in Bodh Gaya before the retreat and had a crush on. Besides those pleasant emotions, I also felt frustration when my body hurt from sitting still and when I could not get my mind to settle on the breath. In those moments, I felt tightness in my jaw and heat rising in my body. And there were moments of feeling inadequate in the practice or of getting caught in wanting—wanting to take a break and walk into the village, wanting to talk to one of my new friends. The display of emotions and the feelings arising were endless. We learned to let go of the storyline that was feeding the emotions and just sit with the feelings, noticing how they arose, changed, and faded away.

The final object of attention that was introduced was the hardest of all. We were asked to pay attention to our thoughts, noticing how they arise, remain for a while, and then vanish. I discovered both how subtle some thoughts were, barely perceptible, and how powerful and overwhelming other thoughts were. We were learning to pay attention to the process of thinking and not to the content of the thoughts, not identifying with them, not getting lost in them, just allowing them to come and go, like clouds in the sky, like leaves passing by in a river.

Mindfully paying attention to my experience, I became increasingly aware of the ongoing flow of body sensations, waves of energy, emotions, thoughts, and mindstates—all changing experiences coming and going. Calm and concentration would be replaced by restlessness and agitation and then return to calm again. Contentment would be replaced by longing and dissatisfaction and then contentment again. No experience lasted. I recognized that the gift mindfulness was offering was not only cultivating moments of joy and calm but also a growing ability to be open and present with all of my experience, without struggle or judgment, no matter what it was. Mindfulness was offering the gift of being at peace with the way things are. I was tasting the peace of returning to an open, spacious, accepting state of being.

Awareness of Breathing and Body Sensations

Begin by finding a comfortable place to sit and set the intention to be awake and aware of your experience moment by moment without judgment. As you take three deep breaths, notice where in your body you predominantly feel the movement of the breath. It may be the feeling of the air as it enters and leaves your nostrils, or maybe the rising and the falling of the abdomen and chest. Notice the changing sensations that arise with each breath. Rest in the movement of the breath. Gradually open your field of awareness to include other sensations in the body. You may feel pressure, tightness, tingling, vibration, itching. As you focus your attention on them, notice how those sensations rise, change, and diminish. When your mind wanders into thought, as it will, gently and without judgment bring your attention back to the movement of the breath. Each time you do this, you are cultivating a deeper connection with yourself. Before returning to your day, give yourself a few moments to notice how your body and mind are feeling after this practice.

As the days of the retreat unfolded, I could feel a growing resonance with the teachings and the practice. Something in me was saying *Yes!* I had actually found what I had been looking for. With that confidence my intention deepened. Often when we find a spiritual path, a teaching, or a practice we resonate with, something about it feels familiar, something about it make sense to us. Our inner wisdom recognizes the wisdom of the practices, our inner truth recognizes the truth of the teachings, the love in our heart meets the love supporting this avenue to freedom. We finally know that there is a way out of self-abandonment and that we are not bound to live our lives stumbling from one moment to the next, perpetuating our suffering. At that retreat I had found that path, and I knew I would follow it back to myself.

Cultivating Intimacy with Our Experience

In one of the stories about Dogen Zenji, the great thirteenth-century Japanese Soto Zen teacher, a student asks him, "What is the awakened mind?" Dogen responds, "The mind that is intimate with all things." He goes on to explain that the Buddhist path of awakening is a path of intimacy, a way of coming close to our experience. Intimacy is the tenderness we feel when we are moved to tears. Intimacy is the closeness and sense of connectedness we feel when our attention rests on the movement of our breath. Intimacy is feeling the tingling of excitement, the warmth of love, or being fully present and alive in our body as we dance or listen to a piece of music that touches us. And intimacy is also our ability to be present for difficult moments, being with the heat of anger, the contraction of fear, or the pain of grief. Intimacy with our experience, whether it is pleasant or unpleasant, is a quality of connection that brings us closer to the truth of each moment.

Mindfulness, awakened attention to our actual experience in the moment, is a practice of intimacy. It supports our journey back to ourselves as we let go of the habit of distancing from our experience and instead cultivate a closeness with ourselves, an interest in who we are. Tim Olmsted, a meditation teacher in the Tibetan tradition, talks about mindfulness as a way of befriending ourselves, an opportunity to spend time with ourselves. When we practice meditation, he says, we get to know ourselves extremely well, we see all parts of ourselves, and we don't turn away. He says that being mindful of our sensations, our thoughts, and our emotions is like hanging out with a good friend for a long time. Over the months and years together, we get to see them for who they are, in all their magnificence and vulnerability. Over time, we grow in affection for this friend, we come to love them, to forgive them, to accept them. In the same way, by being mindful of our experience and getting to know all parts of ourselves, we come to know our own beauty and our vulnerability. We befriend ourselves, forgive ourselves, and grow in affection for ourselves. In other words, we come close to our own unique experience of life, we become intimate with it, and in this way, we take ourselves back into our hearts.

I like to imagine intimacy as the delicacy of two fingers lightly touching each other. This image of touching and being touched evokes feelings of gentleness, tenderness, and safety. In order for such intimacy to arise, we need to slow down, bring our attention to our present experience and rest there, staying long enough to listen to whatever is arising and letting ourselves be touched and affected by it. We might slow down and take in the sweet and sour taste of a freshly picked apple. We might slow down and feel the warmth of a hand we are holding, or the pain in our body and mind when we feel unworthy or lonely. We slow down and, touching and being touched by our experience, we respond with warmth, attentiveness, and care.

Intimacy awakens in us childlike curiosity, the wish to come close, to explore, to know things as they are. We ask ourselves: *What is happening right now? Can I open to it?* This curiosity has been called "beginner's mind," the mind that is open and receptive, with no preconceived ideas of how things should be, just seeing things as they are. We practice with the kind of curiosity we might feel when we travel to a city or country we have never been to before—awake, aware, and engaged in the experience of that new place, we notice the shapes of the buildings, the street signs, the smells and tastes of the local food. Mindfulness practice is about bringing that same curiosity to our inner experience.

Cultivating Intimacy with Our Experience

Find a time when you can be fully present with an activity that gladdens your heart. Let yourself slow down enough to notice the details of your experience—the warmth of the teacup in your hands and the aroma arising from it; the feel of the earth as you tend your garden; the sensation of stretching in a yoga pose, and the flow of warmth as you come out of the stretch; the pleasant sensations of listening to a favorite song or symphony; the colors of the leaves on the trees. Experience each moment with the intimacy of two fingers touching. Before you finish your exploration, set an intention to carry this sense of intimacy into your day, pausing from time to time to remember.

Even when we feel lost and distant from ourselves, instead of wishing that those mindstates would disappear, we gently and carefully bring our attention close to those feelings and get to know them. We may ask ourselves: *Where in my body am I feeling these emotions? What thoughts are arising in my mind?* When we turn to the mindstates and emotions of self-abandonment with curiosity, we get to know them. They are not strangers we fear but feelings we can listen to, attend to, and hold with compassion. When we are intimate with these feelings, we develop trust in our resilience and in our ability to stay with our experience even at difficult times.

When we are mindful and intimate with our experience, we are no longer living one step away from ourselves. We are fully present in and for our life, holding our experience, whatever it is, with an awareness that is as tender and warm, as if we were holding a baby bird in the palm of our hand. Practicing mindfulness is a way of telling ourselves *This moment matters, I care to come close, I care to stay.*

Healing the Pain of the Second Arrow

There is a teaching story in which the Buddha asks a student: If you are struck by an arrow, is it painful? The student of course answers yes, and the Buddha asks: If you are then struck by a second arrow, is it even more painful? In response to the student's nod of agreement, he goes on to explain that when we experience mental and physical pain and judge it as bad or wrong, that is the second arrow. When we are suffering and we tell ourselves there is something wrong with us for being in pain, those judgments are deepening the pain of self-abandonment. The Buddha pointed out that while suffering is inevitable, and we can't always control the "arrows" of pain that come into our lives, instead of adding to our pain by judging ourselves, we can choose to respond with spaciousness and compassion. This is what I thought might help my new client, Ruth, ease the suffering of her depression.

She arrived at my office for her first appointment upset and disheartened. I welcomed her in and gently inquired about what had moved her to seek counseling. She told me she had experienced periodic episodes of depression for most of her adult life. "When these feelings start, it's like a dark blanket coming over me, blotting out everything else. It's hard enough not wanting to get out of bed and not being able to get anything done, but what really hurts are the thoughts that keep putting me down for feeling that way. It's like they're saying, *Why can't you just snap out of it? What's wrong with you? Why can't you be happy like everybody else?*" Ruth burst into tears.

"That sounds so hard, Ruth. It is painful enough to be caught in depression, but those judgmental thoughts are multiplying your suffering." Ruth nodded, wiping her eyes.

"Yes, the depression I can deal with. I have been through these waves many times. I know they will shift, and the heaviness will lift, but those thoughts telling me I am bad for being depressed make it so much worse, and they just don't go away."

I invited Ruth to close her eyes and bring her attention to her body and her mind and see what she was noticing. After a few moments, she said that the sadness felt like a tightness in her throat and the hopelessness like a heavy weight on her chest. "That's what I've been struggling with. And those judgmental voices keep saying, *There you go again, feeling sorry for yourself. What's wrong with you?*"

I decided to tell Ruth the story of the second arrow to give her a way to understand the pain she was in and to open the door to how she could work with it. "The sadness and the hopelessness you feel are the first arrow," I said after I finished the story. "And those condemning voices are the second arrow. Let's work with that second arrow. That voice judging you for being depressed—what does it sound like?"

"It's harsh and loud, like someone yelling at me."

"Is there an image that comes with those feelings?"

Ruth tightened her fists, and it looked like she was folding into herself. "I saw myself holding a whip in my hand, lashing myself for being bad."

"What do you feel when you see that image?"

"My body tightens up and I freeze," she answered.

"Do you think you could put that whip down, Ruth?" I asked gently.

She hesitated. "It's not easy to let go of it," she said. "That voice feels like it is part of me. It's been there for a long time."

"Would you be willing to put it down for just a moment? You can always take it back again."

Ruth nodded. Then as I watched, her fists slowly opened, and one of her hands relaxed on the couch. Her face softened and with a small smile she said, "I did it, I put the whip down. I even feel a little lighter."

As we ended the session, I offered Ruth a practice she could do at home. I knew she had been taking an online mindfulness course and that she could use that as a tool to help ease the pain of her judgmental voices.

"You may want to start your day by setting an intention to hold yourself with loving awareness. And when those painful thoughts come up, instead of getting lost in them, you can stay aware of the sensations you are feeling in your body, just noticing them with mindfulness. You can be mindful of what you are hearing and seeing, what you are smelling or touching, and hold those experiences with a kind awareness. Keeping your attention in the present moment will help you to step away from the harsh voice of the inner judge." Ruth listened attentively and nodded, looking thoughtful as she left my office.

The following week, she arrived for her therapy session with that little smile on her face and told me about the triumph she had felt one evening when she'd managed to be mindful and kind to herself in the midst of depression. "I hadn't slept well the night before, and I could feel the depression settling in," she began. "My heart was heavy, and I felt so sad. All those negative thoughts were coming up again, putting me down for feeling that way. So, I made sure I did everything that needed to get done in the house and then made my way up the stairs. I felt like I was pulling the weight of my body up with each step."

Ruth said she knew she didn't have to believe that scolding voice inside, and if she did, it would only make the depression worse. She remembered our conversation about not following the second arrow but instead staying anchored in her body and holding herself with kind and loving awareness. She said that when she walked into the bathroom, she carefully felt the coolness of the tiles on her bare feet. When she stepped into the shower stall, she felt the smoothness of the faucet as she turned it on. The sound of the flowing water was familiar and calming, and she paid attention to its warmth as it streamed down her back. When those judgmental thoughts arose along with feelings of depression, she felt the salty tears filling her eyes, and she renewed her commitment to not get struck by the second arrow. She kindly returned to the sensations she was experiencing in the moment and held them with loving awareness. As she continued to pay close attention, Ruth noticed that some of the tension in her body was beginning to release. She remained mindful as she turned off the water and reached for the towel. After slowly and mindfully drying herself, she got into bed. Following the sensations of her breath, and holding herself in her heart, she fell asleep.

After listening to Ruth's story, I honored her for the work she had done to free herself from the second arrow. "Now that you have a tool to move your attention away from those judgmental voices, in our next session we can begin to work with the deeper causes of your depression."

Ruth was ready to take that next step. "To stop condemning myself for feeling bad about the depression is at least a beginning. And learning how to hold myself with loving awareness, no matter what, has got to help."

Many of us abandon ourselves when we get lost in the pain of the second arrow, judging ourselves harshly for the feelings of depression, anger, or anxiety. As we saw with Ruth, even when emotions are painful, we can choose to put down the whip and remain present in our body with compassion and loving awareness. At times when the emotional pain and the judgmental thoughts are overwhelming, it can be helpful to turn our attention outward to nature or music, or to spend time with a friend, whatever can give our mind and our heart a place to rest. When we have returned to a calm and stable place within, we can slowly turn back and safely explore those difficult feelings.

Untangling the Tangle

Mindfulness practice brings us back to our experience in the present moment with the intention of freeing us from suffering. Ruth redirected her attention away from overwhelming thoughts and feelings by mindfully focusing on sensations that were neutral or even nurturing. This practice kept her awake and aware and protected her from the swirl of self-judgment and depression. Mindfulness can also free us from suffering when we remain present and observe the difficult thoughts, emotions, and sensations as they arise, allowing them to move through us without getting caught in them. But even after years of practice, staying present in the face of overwhelming feelings can be challenging. This is what happened to me one summer weekend when my husband Ian and I were out camping with friends.

After a refreshing swim at a nearby pond, we began preparations for dinner. The atmosphere was light and easy. I felt relaxed and happy, standing by the picnic table, cutting up fresh baguettes and adding slices of mozzarella cheese and tomatoes from our garden. I carefully drizzled olive oil on each of the small oval sandwiches, added basil leaves and a sprinkle of black pepper. I felt present, mindful, in the moment.

Then I heard Ian's voice ringing out with excitement: "I just got the message. My poems got accepted!" A few months before, we both had responded to the call for submissions for an anthology of poems and short stories written by local authors. Ian, who had been writing poems for years, had sent in a couple of his favorites; I was just beginning to explore creative writing and submitted one of my short stories. A week before, I had received the notice that my story had not been accepted, which wasn't too surprising. It had been a fun and courageous exercise to begin putting my work out in the world, so I felt okay about the rejection notice. At least I thought I did, until the moment of Ian's announcement.

I felt my body tightening up. My thoughts were racing, and angry words started pouring out of my mouth. "No way, no way. There is no way they took both of your poems and didn't take my story." A part of me wanted to rejoice with Ian and celebrate him, but I could not stop those thoughts and feelings. I felt resentful, indignant, jealous, and mad. Our friends, who knew me well, thought at first that I was joking, but it soon became clear that I wasn't. I felt flooded with the pain of rejection.

Many of us may be familiar with that state of getting tangled in painful thoughts and emotions taking over our mind. We may feel hurt by someone and get overwhelmed by waves of anger and blame. Or we may have hurt someone and can't stop the feelings of guilt and regret. We may dwell on the memory of a time when we felt disrespected, humiliated, or shamed. Or we may be overcome by the fear of being abandoned. When we get caught in waves of emotion and powerful stories in our mind, we lose touch with the present moment. We lose touch with our innate goodness, and we forget we can trust ourselves and the people around us. How do we turn back again, how do we "untangle this tangle"?

A story of the Buddha addresses this question of how we can free ourselves from the stories and reactions we get caught in. When he was teaching at a well-known monastery, a man arrived, bowed, and took a place in the front row. When he had a chance, the man urgently asked: "A tangle within, a tangle without, people are entangled in a tangle. Gotama, I ask you this: Who can untangle this tangle?" The Buddha answered that a person who is established in virtue and is mindful and ardently committed to practice can untangle the tangle.

Recognizing with mindfulness that we are caught in a tangle is how we begin turning back. We see clearly that we are lost in a story; we notice the repetitive thoughts running through our mind; we notice waves of emotion rising within us and the unpleasant sensations arising in our body. Instead of getting lost in the thoughts and feelings, we turn toward them with mindful awareness, noticing and exploring our experience: *These are thoughts arising and passing. These are emotions and sensations.*

This is my breath. Remaining mindful, the tangle begins to untangle. We see our thoughts and emotions arise, change, and pass away and we stay centered and grounded, anchored in awareness.

But when we are caught in the tangle, mindfulness can seem far away. That day, when we were out camping, my mind continued spinning the story of rejection. I judged myself for feeling jealous, not an image of myself I wanted to uphold, but I couldn't get out of those feelings. I tried to distract myself by starting to build a fire so we could cook, but the wood was wet. All I got was smoke, a good metaphor for my mindstate. One of our friends asked if I wanted help, but I brushed him off. Not knowing what to do, I dropped into the folding chair by the smoldering wood and just let the thoughts and feelings wash over me. *No way that he got accepted and I didn't. This is not okay.* A small voice whispered, *What about me?* Even in the midst of that feeling of righteousness, I could see that I was caught. Repeating the story was not freeing me from the tangle, it was only making the knot tighter.

At some point I noticed myself taking a deep breath. My many years of mindfulness practice arose for me in that moment. I brought my attention inward and carefully observed the emotions as they manifested as sensations. Jealousy appeared as tightness in my chest, anger and resentment as waves of heat rising through the center of my body. I repeated to myself, *Just observe, just be with this without judgment.*

After about fifteen minutes of paying mindful attention to these feelings, the waves of emotion began to subside, and the urge to fight left my body. The following moments of quiet made room for more tender emotions to arise. I noticed a pulsating ache in my chest along with a feeling of vulnerability. Holding these sensations with gentle awareness allowed something in me to soften. The tightness in my chest released and I felt ready to open my eyes. When I looked up, I could see the flames dancing and smell the delicious vegetables that were being cooked on the grill.

Feeling centered and grounded, I stood up, walked over to Ian, and said, "I guess those feelings were buried for the last few days, and all it took was hearing about your poems to bring them out. I am truly happy for you." He held me gently as my heart opened again.

As I later reflected on what had happened by the campfire, I could see that the feelings of not being included, of not being welcomed, that came up that evening were not new. A memory arose of a time when I was about ten years old, and my friends suddenly stopped talking to me and I had no idea why. Other memories of feeling rejected came to mind—living in Israel and not getting a job I wanted at a peace organization; a time when I applied to participate in a workshop but got turned down. I could still feel in my body the feelings of bewilderment and humiliation at being left out. Over the next few days, I noticed the thoughts, feelings, and sensations accompanying those memories appear in my mind, and as I patiently held them with mindfulness, they released. I was untangling the tangle.

Being *aware* of self-abandonment is significantly different from being *lost* in self-abandonment. When we are mindful of being lost in a painful story or difficult emotions, we can gently and kindly bring our attention back to the body and allow the underlying hurts to be revealed and move through us. As we hold the flow of sensation and emotions with mindfulness, the tangle unwinds.

With wisdom and compassion, we can discern and choose the ways we use mindfulness to free ourselves from difficult mindstates. When our experience is overwhelming and we find ourselves lost in stories of the past or lost in judgment, like Ruth, we can use mindfulness to redirect our attention to pleasant and neutral sensations. This allows us to regroup and re-establish a calm and steady attention in the present moment. We can also use mindfulness as I did, remaining present with difficult thoughts, emotions, and sensations as they move through us. Instead of getting caught in reacting, avoiding, fighting with, or judging our experience, we turn toward it, open to it, and hold it with a loving awareness. With mindfulness we cultivate equanimity, our ability to remain balanced, nonreactive, and spacious when suffering arises.

Mindfulness strengthens our trust in ourselves and gives us the heart to be present with both joy and sorrow. It supports our ability to turn to our pain and hold it with kindness. Awake and aware, we flow between these two ways of practicing mindfulness, both keeping us in the present moment.

Everyday Mindfulness

"It is not hard to be mindful, it is hard to remember to be mindful." This insightful observation by Joseph Goldstein, the co-founder of the Insight Meditation Society (IMS) in Barre, Massachusetts, and one of the leading insight meditation teachers in the West, sums up something we easily notice every day. When we are rushing about or multitasking, it is easy to get lost in "doing" and lose touch with our inner experience in the moment. We might be cooking dinner, helping our children with their homework, and trying to remember what we will need to prepare for work tomorrow, all at the same time. In the midst of the pots, the math problems, and the calendar, it is hard to remember to be mindful of our body, our thoughts, and our feelings. Or on a busy morning, we might take a shower, get dressed, and be on our way to work before we realize that we've not been mindful since we got out of bed. Carried away by memories of the past or lost in thoughts of an imagined future, mindfulness is the last thing on our mind.

When my daughter Tamar was four months old, I returned to working part-time as a physical therapist. Our trustworthy neighbor Crow came in to care for her, and even though I missed my baby, at work I felt present and centered. But one day for no apparent reason, as I was driving home, I suddenly found myself feeling anxious, my entire focus narrowed down to one thought: *I need to get to Tamar!!!* It felt like my life depended on it. I've come to call that feeling "the pull in my tummy," the mother instinct of needing to defend her offspring that pushes everything else out of the way. At that moment I was no longer in touch with my body. I wasn't seeing the bright blue sky or the shimmering colors of the fall leaves on the trees. I was utterly un-mindful, caught up in fear and self-judgment: *I should never have gone back to work. I should have stayed home with Tamar like some of my other friends with new babies.*

Caught in that swirl of emotion, I arrived home, jumped out of the car, threw open the front door, and dashed into the living room. There was Tamar, peacefully shaking a rattle, listening to Crow play guitar. While I was relieved and delighted to see that my baby was safe and happy, I also felt deflated. It was clear to me that I had lost myself to anxiety, worry, and self-judgment. With a small tear at the corner of my eye, I sat down on the rug and watched my little girl, contemplating the contrast between this sweet, calm scene and my frenzy.

Puzzled by my overreaction, I reached out to Myoshin Kelley, an insight meditation teacher and friend. I described to her the ride home, being consumed by anxiety, and the sense of self-abandonment I felt. Her instruction was simple: "Don't try to be ahead of yourself. Use the drive home each day as your meditation. Stay close to your experience, stay in the moment." I was being called to practice mindfulness in the midst of my daily life.

After that, each day when I was leaving work, I tried to remember to slow down and be present before starting the car. I reminded myself to feel the touch of my hands on the steering wheel, to feel my breath. There was one specific day when I felt the "pull in my tummy" again and the urgency to get home. With Myoshin's teaching in my mind, I used that moment as my meditation. First, I noticed that my whole body was leaning forward, and I told myself to settle back into my seat and take a breath. I had to do that several times during the drive. I noticed I was having conversations with traffic lights, getting upset at them for not changing to green fast enough. I had to laugh at myself for that one, and seeing clearly the way my mind was reacting helped me ease into the moment. The rest of the drive I managed to be mostly present.

When I arrived home, this time I was able to graciously thank Crow, and I carried Tamar up to our bedroom for a nap. We lay together on the bed, the warmth of her little body against mine, the afternoon light filling the space. Her silky hair felt soft as my fingers stroked her head. Any remnants of anxiety from the rush home had dissipated, and I relaxed into the simplicity of being together. My heart was filled with gratitude for the preciousness of that moment. I listened to her breath and noticed mine. Bathed in appreciation, my mind was not wandering or planning. Settled into my body, my eyelids grew heavy, and we slept side by side.

How do we cultivate mindfulness in daily life? How do we remember to be mindful? Practicing mindfulness in a dedicated way, daily or at least several times a week, can certainly help us remember to be present, for it strengthens the inclination of the mind to be awake and aware. It is said that each moment of mindfulness is the seed of the next, and so the more we practice, the more moments of mindfulness spontaneously arise. I have found that starting my day with meditation, even ten or fifteen minutes of intentionally paying attention to my body and mind, sets the tone for the rest of my day and allows me to be more present, more kind, and less reactive throughout.

You might say, "I have no time to slow down, I work five days a week, I wake up at 5:30 in the morning and get home at 8 or 9 at night. I am on the go all the time." When taking time out of our day for dedicated meditation practice is not possible, we can practice being present in the midst of our activities. We do not need to be still in a meditation posture to be mindful. We can practice mindfulness when we walk down the street, feeling our steps on the sidewalk and listening to the sound of the birds, or the sound of traffic. We can practice mindfulness while we are chopping vegetables for dinner or when we do the dishes. In the midst of our daily life, we are called to be awake and aware—that is where our practice happens.

Off-the-Cushion Mindfulness Meditation

Choose an activity you perform daily. It may be preparing dinner, putting on your shoes, or brushing your teeth. This can be your off-the-cushion practice. Set the intention to use this time as an act of kindness to yourself. Begin your practice by pausing and bringing your attention to your body. As you do your task, notice the sensations of touch. Notice what you are seeing, smelling, or tasting. What sounds accompany your actions? Notice when your mind wanders, and gently return to mindful attention with gratitude for the gift of the moment.

With dedication to our mindfulness practice, we grow in our ability to be intimately present for the ever-changing flow of body sensations, thoughts, and emotions. We see waves of energy rise and subside, moods come and go, many thoughts moving through our field of awareness, and we stay, not turning against ourselves no matter what arises. We learn to untangle the tangle, to not get caught in stories, thoughts, and beliefs. We learn to not feed negative emotions but instead to remain present in the moment, intimate and curious. There is an ease that comes from abiding in awareness that is open and spacious, not resisting life's endless changes. Over time we develop confidence in our ability to remain awake and aware and to meet the moments of our life with wisdom and grace.

In a very real and direct way, mindfulness protects us from falling into self-abandonment. When we are mindful, we know when we have strayed off the path and we can turn back to ourselves. Resting in loving awareness, we listen to ourselves and to the world around us and respond with kindness. We move lightly on the Earth, not harming life out of carelessness. Being mindful opens the path for the wise and compassionate self to manifest in the world.

Chapter Three

Taking Ourselves Back into Our Hearts: Turning Back with Compassion

I had left Israel as a girl with a backpack and dreams about mountains, beaches, and a curiosity about meditation, and I returned as a changed young woman looking at the world through a new spiritual lens. When I tried to reconnect with old friends, I saw how different I was now. Some of my friendships survived the change, others dropped away. Many of those I'd been closest to were getting married and starting their own families. Once again, I felt I did not fit in.

Despite being introduced to the benefits of mindfulness, I still felt lonely and craved intimacy with others. I kept falling in love with one man after another, projecting my longing for wholeness and fulfillment onto each of them, hoping that being loved by them would make me happy. What I still didn't know was that the deep longing I felt was for a meaningful loving relationship with myself. After several years of going to college in Israel and trying to settle back into my life there, the sense of unease persisted, and the only thing that felt right was to continue exploring the meditation practice I had learned in India.

I set out for Asia again and made my way back to Bodh Gaya. Arriving in the village and walking around the grounds of the Mahabodhi Temple, I felt like I was coming home. I had a sense of belonging among the other spiritual seekers gathered to participate in the annual Vipassana retreat being held at the Thai temple. On the opening day of the retreat there, I knew what to expect. I looked forward to the practice, the rituals, and the flow of the day. I trusted the Dharma to help me find my way back from the emotional pain of loneliness and separation I was carrying. By the time those ten days were over, I knew that all I wanted to do was continue this inner journey.

When I heard about an upcoming three–month meditation retreat at IMS something clicked. Three whole months of silence seemed both daunting and attractive. There was no question about whether I would do it, but it took some time for that dream to manifest. I participated in several more retreats, and then the day arrived. I was standing at the bottom of the steps in front of IMS, in Barre, Massachusetts, on the opening day of the course. *Could I really do it? Spend three months in silence, meditating?* I stood there with my two small bags, containing all they'd said I would need for those months. I took a deep breath and looked up. Above the entrance was the word "Metta," lovingkindness in Pali. That is what my heart was longing for. *Could I find it here?* My heart beating, I took a deep breath, walked up the steps, opened the door, and entered, ready to embark on this next phase of my journey. The many stories I had heard about this place from the teachers I studied with in Bodh Gaya were about to take shape and form for me.

The building was large and old, very different from the Thai temple in Bodh Gaya, but the feeling of deep quiet and welcome was similar. All around me meditation practitioners were meeting up with old friends, hugging and smiling. As I found my way to my room, I heard clatter from the kitchen, where the staff was preparing our first meal. Small notes everywhere were telling us how to take care of ourselves while we were in silence for those three months. I dropped my bags on the bed I had been assigned and went exploring. The dining room and the downstairs room where we would be doing walking meditation were places I had only seen in my imagination, and now here they were, appearing before my eyes. I was here at last.

That evening as I entered the meditation hall, my steps immediately slowed down. My attention dropped into my body and my breath deepened as I felt the touch of my feet on the cool hardwood floor. I recognized the familiar feeling of entering the sacred space a retreat offers. I was ready to begin again.

As the days unfolded, I relaxed ever more deeply into mindfulness practice, bringing my attention back to the present moment again and again, receiving my experience with kindness. But soon all the ways I had been distracting myself from seeing patterns of self-abandonment—staying busy, working, traveling, struggling in relationships, moving from apartment to apartment—were no longer there to protect me. I began noticing the stream of judgmental thoughts. *I am not making enough effort. I have to try harder. I'm taking too much food in the lunch line. I'm eating too fast.* That voice inside compared me to other meditators—some days I was better than them, other days worse. My mind was consumed by wanting connection to others, wanting to be seen and appreciated, wanting something outside of myself that would make me happy. I tried to be mindfully aware of those thoughts and not cling to them, but they arose over and over.

Eventually I began noticing the emotions that were underlying those thoughts. The moments of calm and delight in the practice were often overshadowed by the pain of self-judgment and longing for love. I became intimate with loneliness, anxiety, and an underlying level of what felt like mild depression. As instructed, I observed these emotions in their naked form, as sensations in my body—an ache in my chest, fluttering sensations in my stomach, at times a heaviness that weighed me down. Some of these feelings were very familiar, but in the silence of the retreat they felt amplified. I couldn't avoid seeing them clearly and feeling them intensely. I felt vulnerable, with nowhere to hide. My heart longed for something to ease my inner struggle and help me hold onto a sense of well-being.

The teachers understood that in the silence of the retreat we were seeing the thoughts and beliefs about ourselves that were keeping us from being happy, and that in the face of the truth of our suffering, we were feeling tender and vulnerable. To soothe and uplift us, they introduced the four *Brahma Viharas,* the "Divine Abodes." Lovingkindness, compassion, sympathetic joy, and equanimity were taught by the Buddha as doorways to the heart. Lovingkindness, *Metta* in Pali, arises from seeing the beauty in ourselves and others, and with unconditional friendliness and unconditional love, offers wishes of well-being. Compassion, *Karuna* in Pali, is the quality of heart that turns toward the pain in ourselves and others and holds it with tenderness and care. Sympathetic joy, *Mudita,* is the experience of the heart rejoicing in the joy of others and letting that joy uplift and multiply our own. And equanimity, *Upekkha,* is the quality of the heart that deeply cares and yet remains balanced and centered, holding suffering without getting caught in it nor pushing it away.

As the teachers explained, cultivating these four states of mind is a way to heal and bridge the sense of separation we feel from ourselves and others. These beautiful qualities, each in their own way, slowly erode the walls around our heart and open us to love and compassion for all living beings. *Could that be possible for me?* I wondered. I felt drawn to the promise of these practices.

Each night after giving a talk and guiding a meditation, the teachers ended the evening by chanting the traditional metta phrases in Pali. Radiating love and compassion, they wished us to be happy and free from pain and suffering. The protective walls around my heart would soften and my heart would break open, uncovering an ocean of grief. As tears rolled down my cheeks, I could feel the difficult emotions I had encountered during the day dissolve and release. I felt as if I were being held by a kind mother who loved me, saw my pain, and made room for me in her heart. During those meditation periods, the harsh voices of self-judgment, self-hatred, and self-doubt momentarily would subside. Being held lovingly by the teachers transformed the pain of isolation into a profound sense of connectedness and belonging, the recognition that I was part of a larger whole.

But while I could take in the love radiating from the teachers, when the practice of sending metta to ourselves was introduced, I hit a wall inside. One afternoon, Sharon Salzberg, a lead teacher at the retreat and co-founder of IMS, gently guided us in learning lovingkindness practice. We begin, she said, by reflecting on our own beautiful qualities and our wholesome deeds, and then sending ourselves wishes for happiness and well-being. I repeated the words silently—*May I be happy. May I be peaceful. May I be free from pain and suffering*—but my heart felt like a rock, hardened by all those times I'd felt lonely, different, like I did not belong. I loved what Sharon was saying about the practice, and I wanted my heart to open so I could receive the lovingkindness I was trying to offer myself, but I was unable to feel the warmth I felt when the teachers sent us metta. Directing the phrases to myself, the words felt empty and hollow. Right there in those moments of struggle, unable to love myself, I clearly knew the experience of self-abandonment.

I felt so discouraged, and in one of my weekly meetings with Sharon, I shared my struggle. Sharon kindly reassured me that coming up against such barriers was part of the practice, and she encouraged me to stay with it and trust my intention to open my heart to myself. Being in her presence I could feel the warmth of metta wash over me, but when I returned to my meditation cushion, the wall was up again.

Then one night Michele McDonald, another of the teachers, gave a talk about challenges she had encountered in her own practice. She told us that when she first learned the Brahma Viharas, she found it a struggle to feel love for herself. I nodded. *Yes, I get it.* Her heart softened, she said, when she began practicing the second Brahma Vihara, compassion, holding the pain in her heart with love. I felt a sense of relief.

I was not failing in the practice. I could turn to myself with compassion. That would be the key for me to begin opening my heart.

That night Michele taught us the practice of compassion. Acknowledging that we are hurting, we say: *May I open my heart to my pain, May I open my heart to my sorrow.* In doing so we honor our wish to be free of suffering. With these words the warmth and caring of compassion gently entered my heart.

In Buddhist texts, *karuna* literally means the quivering of the heart in response to suffering. I spent the rest of the retreat holding my painful experiences with a quivering heart, tenderly touching my deep longings and my vulnerability, meeting my suffering with kindness. Compassion does not resist the pain we are experiencing, nor does it judge that pain. Rather, it turns toward the pain, comes close to the suffering, and holds it with warmth, patience, and care. With compassion we learn to turn to ourselves with kindness and love, trusting in the wisdom of the practice to free us from suffering.

We might ask ourselves, why would we even want to open our heart to pain? Why not just find ways to cope with or get around the difficulties in our lives? That strategy might be nice if it worked, but in the First Noble Truth the Buddha proclaims that suffering is unavoidable—something we all know. On our journey through life, we all face the demons of greed, hatred, and delusion; we all walk through dark forests and sail through stormy seas. Pain is part of the fabric of our life, and turning toward it with an open heart can call forth from within us the warmth of compassion that allows us to be with suffering without shutting down, without abandoning ourselves. Compassion allows us to hold our suffering with courage and love.

We all encounter those times when we feel lost, distant from ourselves, and unable to hold our pain with love. But when we gently and carefully turn toward these vulnerable feelings and meet them with understanding and compassion, the way we would hold a child who is hurting, we can begin to find our way back to our heart.

Finding Compassion in a True Other

As the three-month retreat was drawing to a close, I knew that something in me had changed. At times I had experienced the freedom and ease that came from letting go of self-judgment and attachment, and at times I had experienced the joy and beauty of insight and understanding. And at times I remembered to hold my suffering with compassion. But those months of meditation had also dissolved the barriers I had put up. I no longer had the shield I had carried before to protect myself from the pain inside. I had set out on the journey of healing the heart, but now that the retreat was ending, I didn't know what the next steps could possibly be.

Feeling raw and vulnerable, I went for a final check-in with Sharon and to say goodbye. With obvious concern and great kindness, she said, "I have been thinking about you. I noticed your shoulders trembling during the late-night meditations, and I know it has not been an easy retreat for you." Tears welled up again as I told her, "I have been crying for the last three days. My heart feels wide open and there is so much pain." To my surprise she said, "You might want to work with a therapist." While Sharon understood the value of silent retreats, she also knew that turning toward our pain can sometimes be more than a daily meditation practice can handle. Immersing myself in deep meditation practice had exposed the pain of self-abandonment I'd been carrying. Following Sharon's guidance, I would reach out for a healing relationship with a professional counselor. That would be a critical part of finding my way back to my heart.

Turning to others for support can be challenging for some of us, especially if we have been dismissed, let down, or disappointed when we previously sought help. Some may believe that reaching for support is a sign of weakness or fear, making themselves vulnerable by revealing the pain in their heart in therapy, and so they hold their pain close to their heart, not sharing it with others. But hitting a low and painful point in our lives, recognizing that we can no longer continue doing what we have been doing for months or years, can be the benevolent push that gets us over the threshold and into trusting the care of others. I was ready for that at last.

After getting a visa that would allow me to live and work in the United States, I found a place to live in the town of Barre, about a mile down the road from IMS. Even though I had been living in the States before, I felt like I was in an unfamiliar land. I was living alone in a small, funky apartment during an especially cold and snowy winter. Being used to a warm climate with very mild winters, I found driving on the icy roads challenging and scary. Still, several nights a week I drove over to IMS to listen to Dharma talks. But the meditators were in silence, and the staff were involved in their own lives, so I didn't really feel part of the community.

There was one saving grace. I got a job working in an Early Intervention program, providing physical therapy to infants and toddlers with developmental delays. I drove from house to house to visit the children, carrying with me a large therapy ball and a bag full of toys. I enjoyed stepping into the warm homes where people were happy to see me. One mother greeted me each week with a cup of hot tea and freshly baked muffins. She'd ask me about my life, wanting to know how it felt to be living in a foreign country. Those moments of warmth and care reminded me of the connection I was longing for.

But returning to my empty apartment night after night brought me right to my edge and amplified the pain I had opened to on the three-month retreat. Trying to meditate didn't seem to be helping, and before too long, loneliness and depression took over. Remembering Sharon's advice, I finally started looking for a therapist.

Diana Fosha speaks of what she calls "unbearable aloneness," the distress we feel when we are confronted with overwhelming physical and emotional pain without support. She points out that this form of aloneness is different from the spiritual aloneness and solitude we might deliberately seek out as part of the journey back to ourselves. Rather, this is what someone experiences when they are utterly alone with no one to talk to. As a trauma therapist, she points out that this is especially impactful for those who have experienced neglect or abuse, but even for those not facing that level of traumatic experience, being alone and isolated can lead to this feeling of "unbearable aloneness," of being utterly on our own in the world, lost in self–abandonment. When we find ourselves feeling hopeless and unable to find our way back to ourselves, the most compassionate and loving thing we can do is to connect with what Diana Fosha calls a "true other." She defines the true other as a caring, supportive person who holds us in kind and tender regard and can open the door for us to love and accept ourselves. For me, that "true other" would be Carol.

Carol lived a couple of towns away from my apartment. One afternoon, feeling hesitant and slightly shivering, though not from the cold, I walked down the snowy path leading to her house for our first visit. There, next to the door, I was met by a stone statue of Quan Yin, the Buddhist goddess of mercy and compassion. That image of caring and support gave me the courage to knock on the door and once again step into the unknown. Carol greeted me with a warm and welcoming smile. "Come on in, make yourself comfortable," she said as she took my coat and hung it on an ornate wooden stand. "Were the roads not too icy today?" she inquired. I felt immediately at ease. Carol was motherly and loving. I felt safe in her presence and knew I could trust her wisdom and skill to take me on the journey of emotional healing that would allow me to take myself back into my heart.

Week after week Carol met me with compassion. She listened to my stories and witnessed my tears with tenderness and kindness. She took a sincere interest in my life and validated my feelings. "It makes sense to me that you would feel lonely living by yourself in the small town of Barre," she said at our first meeting. "Of course you are missing your family." When I'd tell her about something difficult I had experienced, she would say with understanding, "I'm so sorry you had to go through all that—it sounds so confusing." In Carol's presence I felt protected, safe, and understood. I could let down my guard and be vulnerable. She held me with compassion as waves of grief moved through me, not judging, not blaming, not trying to take the pain away. Her caring response to my stories softened the voices inside that were asking: *What's wrong with me? Why I am holding onto relationships that aren't working? Why is meditation not working for me? Why can't I pull myself out of this by myself?* Carol's message of compassion was: "Yes, this is hard, and you are not alone. I will help you get through this." Carol became an anchor in my life, a place to rest, relax, and replenish. With her support, I no longer needed to figure out my life by myself. With her by my side, even the cold winter now seemed bearable.

Held in the Compassion of a True Other

Call to mind the image of someone who supported you at a time when you were hurting—maybe a family member, a dear friend, or a counselor you have worked with. It might be a spiritual being, an angel, Quan Yin, or the Virgin Mary. As you recall that memory of being held in the compassion of a true other, what do you feel in your body? What do you feel in your heart? How did the presence of that being help you move through that challenging time in your life? When you are ready, bring your attention back to the present moment and allow gratitude to arise for the presence of that being in your life. Let yourself carry the sense of being supported and cared for throughout your day.

Yet at times Carol's compassion could be very clear and direct. Whenever I fell into the habits of self-abandonment, she would help me see that and bring me back to myself. For example, for several weeks I came to her caught up in trying to hang onto what was essentially a lost-cause love interest. She didn't hesitate to call me on it. "Each time you reach out to Tom, it's like an alcoholic reaching out for another drink. Hold yourself back from phoning him or going to his house, and bring your emotions to our session instead. Together we can work on the feelings that are coming up." Kindly but firmly, she encouraged me to turn back to myself. I sometimes kicked and screamed inside, but I had to admit that her wisdom was guiding me away from suffering and toward happiness.

Finding the Source of Compassion Within

Being in the presence of a compassionate other gives us the safety, strength, and courage to turn toward the pain that is asking for loving attention. As we open our heart to receive compassion from others, we begin to connect with the source of compassion within ourselves. This is what I was learning with Carol. In her caring presence, I began to remember the many times in my life when I had been held with love and compassion. When I was a child, my father was the "doctor" in the house, tending to us when we scraped our knees falling off our bicycles, climbing trees, or playing soccer. I'd follow him into the bathroom, sit down, and wait while he filled a small basin with warm water. He'd dip a washcloth in and gently squeeze the water over the wound, loosening the dirt, washing away the blood, and soothing the sting and pain and upset. I clearly remember the pungent smell of the antiseptic wash, an orange-brown liquid that turned white in water. It looked like some magical alchemical process. Then, with great care, he'd take gauze and a topical, thick, pink ointment and cover the sore. I'd count to ten until the burning sensation subsided. My father never got angry at us for falling; he never shamed us for getting hurt. Instead, he took *care* of us, in the truest meaning of that word. Thinking back, I no longer remember the pain of the scrape, but I clearly remember the experience of being held in compassion.

Working with Carol, I also remembered how my mother listened to me with tender care when my heart was hurting. One night stands out. I was twelve or thirteen years old and had just watched a movie about the Vietnam War. I was overcome with sadness by the magnitude of suffering I had just witnessed. I was especially moved by the care the female nurses in the film were providing to the wounded. I felt within me a strong urge to do something to stop the pain in the world. I wanted to do what those nurses were doing, but I was young and didn't know how to go about it. My mother heard me crying and came into my room. She sat down next to me on my bed, a faint stream of light entering from the hallway. With her hand resting on my leg, she listened with care, allowing the feelings to move through me, not trying to give advice or solve the problem but trusting that just being with me would help me find my way back to calm. When the waves of sadness passed, we spoke for a long time. She listened, affirming the surge of compassion that had arisen within me. She then tucked me in, kissed me good night, and put out the light. Recalling those memories, I appreciated the seeds of compassion that had been planted in me. As I felt the warmth in my heart and gratitude for my parents' love, and I recognized that I was worthy of their love, I began to open my heart to myself.

About a year into my ongoing sessions with Carol, I began to feel put together again. The depression lifted, my body started to feel stronger, and even my heart felt a little lighter. In Carol's compassionate presence, I could see the seeds of self–love beginning to sprout, but it would take another important step with her before they could begin to blossom into abiding compassion for myself.

One afternoon after I had once again shared a story of heartbreak and loneliness and shed many tears, with a kind look in her eyes, Carol said, "You have cried enough, Dalya. Let's try something different." Slightly taken aback by this change in her approach, I paused. I was reluctant to let go of being the lonely young woman in a strange country, feeling sad and sorry for myself. But by that time, I had come to trust Carol, so I sat back ready to listen.

She asked me to close my eyes and call to mind a time when I had felt in touch with what she called "the centered self." This part of the self, she said, has the qualities of wisdom and compassion. Almost immediately an image arose in my mind of an evening in Israel when I led a meditation for a group of friends. I remembered feeling centered, confident, and calm. As I held the memory in mind, I felt myself automatically adjusting my posture, sitting taller, confidently taking my place in the world with a heart full of compassion. The heaviness in my chest that I had been feeling just minutes before lifted. I felt fully present. I had met my centered self.

"Now can you turn to this centered self and ask her to offer compassion to the parts of yourself that have been hurting?" As I did so, I had the sense of connecting to Quan Yin inside me, to Sharon and Carol inside me, and to my parents. Just as I had received compassion from them, I knew that I now could offer that to myself. Carol asked me to rest in that centered self and from that place inside to listen to the parts of myself that were hurting, not judging or rejecting any of them, just hearing what they had to say and holding them with compassion and kindness. After a few minutes she asked me to put my hand on my heart and quietly say, "I care about myself." This was one of the same phrases I had heard from Michele at IMS when I first learned the compassion practice. I closed my eyes and, with my hand on my heart, slowly spoke the words. After repeating the phrase for a couple of minutes, I could begin to feel the tension leaving my body and warmth rising in my chest. As I continued, I could feel the warmth of compassion for myself deepen. And now, after all my work with Carol to release the pain that had made me close my heart, I was at last able to take in the care I was offering myself. As we completed the session, Carol said, "Now that you know how to hold yourself with kindness, Dalya, please call on your centered self when you are sad or lonely. Invite that quality of compassion to come with you wherever you are."

On our journey back to ourselves there is a point that feels magical when we reconnect to the wellspring of love, wisdom, and compassion within us. We shift out of being the victim of our upbringing, out of being lost in self-abandonment, and we find ourselves touching the place inside us that knows we are worthy of love, that knows we belong in the world. That is what I had experienced with Carol, an inner strength that made me feel tall and centered and at the same time grounded and connected to the earth; a strength that let me hold myself with love and compassion. Although that connection would need to be practiced and strengthened, I now knew a place within myself I could always return to.

For months after that session, I drove through the Massachusetts countryside with one hand on the steering wheel and one hand on my heart, reciting the compassion phrase, *I care about myself.* I repeated it softly over and over, and I began to feel cared for, not by someone else but by compassion itself. I felt as if I were in the company of compassion as my "true other." The waves of loneliness and depression I had carried for so long were diminishing, making room for love, joy, and connection with others.

No matter what the cause of our pain, at times we need to receive compassion from others before we can give it to ourselves. Those compassionate others might be teachers, friends, parents, a counselor or mentor—someone who understands us, holds us in love, and is willing to offer us their presence and wisdom as we take ourselves back into our hearts. Reaching out for that support is a brave and compassionate act, a gift we can then give ourselves on our journey.

Calling on the Source of Compassion Within

When you find yourself facing the pain of difficult thoughts and emotions, you can call on the source of compassion in yourself to support you. Take a moment to notice what you are feeling in your body, your mind and heart. Then let yourself remember a time when you experienced a heartfelt sense of confidence, a time when you felt centered and trusted yourself, when you felt connected to the source of wisdom and compassion within you. Now, from that place, turn to the pain you are feeling and listen with kindness. With a hand on your heart, offer yourself the words of compassion: "I care about myself," or "May I open my heart to myself without fear and without judgment." Continue offering yourself the phrases of compassion, trusting that over time warmth and caring will enter your heart.

Learning the Practice of Compassion

A number of years after working with Carol, I started leading meditation circles for women. By that time, I was living in Upstate New York, was married to Ian, and had settled into a new life. The meaningful healing I had found in my work with Carol had shown me the importance of having the presence and witness of supportive others, and I wanted to offer that to my community. My wish was to create a space for women to engage in intimate and truthful conversation, to draw upon the clarity of mindfulness, and to relate to themselves with lovingkindness and compassion, greater self-acceptance, and greater joy.

One evening I received a phone call from a woman who had heard about the circle. Even in her first few words I could hear her voice trembling. With a kind of desperation, Colleen launched into telling me about the upheaval happening in her life. Several months prior, she had moved in with her boyfriend, Jacob, and now they seemed to be arguing almost every day. She could barely recognize the person she had become. Feeling angry and ashamed, she said she was willing to do anything it would take to return to feeling more like herself, like the person she was when she and Jacob fell in love. "The weakest muscle in my body is my mind," she said in tears. "I don't know how to calm down. I don't seem to know how to be kind to myself ... or to anyone else. I have been struggling with this for so long now. I thought talking with other women and learning meditation in your group might help."

"We meet once a month on Sunday mornings. If that would work for you, Colleen, why don't you come this week?"

When she arrived for her first meeting, I noticed her nervously scanning the room as she looked for a place to sit. During the opening circle, she told us she was there because she was struggling with her relationship. But it would take a couple more meetings before she felt comfortable enough to begin telling us more about herself.

Slowly revealing her story, our hearts were touched with compassion. Colleen told us she had grown up in a chaotic home, the second of four siblings. Her mother had a volatile temper and, because she suffered from an autoimmune disease, was not available for the children most of the time. When she did get out of bed, she was often angry and always unpredictable. Colleen's father, who was recovering from a mental breakdown, spent most evenings after work drinking, eventually falling asleep in his recliner chair in front of the TV. Colleen survived the chaos by trying not to draw attention to herself and doing what was expected of her. She folded the laundry, swept the floors, washed the dishes. She often stayed home from school to keep her mother company and do housework. With a little smile, Colleen told us she'd often thought of herself as Cinderella, waiting for her fairy godmother to come to the rescue.

In high school her music teacher did become that fairy godmother. Recognizing Colleen's talent, she reached out and offered support, often staying after school to talk with her, and eventually helped her get into a good college where she could study the arts. There Colleen discovered a new life and ended up spending her twenties living in the company of artists, discovering her creativity, her joy and aliveness, and not thinking much about her past. But when she moved in with Jacob and found herself back in a "close family" situation, the patterns and memories of her abusive childhood came roaring back. She felt trapped and desperate, fighting to hold onto the alive and creative person she had become.

"I know it's not anything Jacob is doing," Colleen said, "but I just can't seem to keep from lashing out at him. Our life has become a battlefield."

She told us that enormous waves of anger would move through her, brought on by the slightest annoyance. At first, she had enjoyed the power she felt in speaking her truth to Jacob, not holding back or being silent as she had to do when she was a child. But she had begun to see the emotional devastation left behind by her rage. She saw the fear in his eyes and watched him shut down and retreat. She knew that when she exploded in anger or stomped out of the house, she was abandoning not only Jacob but also herself.

When Colleen concluded her story, she covered her face and sobbed. I moved over and sat by her side, quietly saying, "Let's breathe together." As her breath gradually deepened, I asked her to open her eyes and look around the room. "Notice the faces of all of us here with you." As Colleen paused to connect with each woman, her eyes filled with tears again, as the love and compassion emanating from the women in the room held her tenderly.

"Thank you for listening to me," Colleen said softly. "I haven't told my story to many people in my life. It is such a relief to be listened to and not hold it by myself." In the love and compassionate presence of the women in the circle, Colleen had found a "true other." Being heard and accepted for who she was, a layer of shame had been peeled away. Feeling seen as more than just an angry unhappy woman, she would begin finding her way back to that loving and alive person she knew she could be.

But then a couple of months later, during her check-in, the fear and agitation Colleen had first told us about was back again. She and Jacob had just learned they were expecting a child. Panicked, Colleen said, "I don't know how to be in a loving relationship with Jacob let alone know how to relate to a baby in a way that could possibly be good for it." Her body was shaking as she told us how scared and confused she felt. She was two months pregnant and was struggling to sleep at night and had started feeling nauseous most of the time. "I can smell the stench of the garbage truck even when it's a few streets away," she told us, "and the smell of certain foods is intolerable."

Several other women in the group were mothers and could well understand the upheaval pregnancy could bring, especially in the midst of relationship challenges. Everyone was clearly moved by Colleen's situation, and I could see this would be a good time to introduce self-compassion as a way to hold the kind of pain Colleen was facing.

I began by saying that, as the Buddha taught, we all wish to be happy, but all of us experience physical, emotional, or mental pain at different times in our life. "With the tender understanding that we all suffer and that we are not alone in experiencing pain, we can offer compassion to ourselves and to each other as a balm for the heart." I suggested that they settle comfortably into their seats.

"As you are aware of all of us together in the circle today, you might notice the warmth of compassion connecting us to each other. Let's breathe in that warmth." After a minute or so, I said, "Now allow your attention to turn inward and ask yourself if there is anything in you that is calling for attention right now." I noticed a tear appearing at the corner of Colleen's eye. After a few moments of silence, I went on:

"If there is anything in your mind and heart that is hurting right now, gently breathe into that. You might place your hand on your heart, and holding yourself with great kindness, let yourself silently repeat these words of compassion: 'May I be free from pain, may I be free from sorrow. May I open my heart to myself without fear and without judgment.' Or you might simply say, 'I care about myself.'" I could sense the depth of compassion each woman in the group was offering herself. I ended the meditation by suggesting that they send that feeling of warmth and care to each other.

When the meditation was over, Colleen looked calm. "This was a new experience for me," she told us. "I had never before thought of holding myself with kindness and having compassion for all those negative feelings. But something happened in that meditation. For a few minutes I actually did start feeling some compassion for myself and everything that's going on with me right now."

As we closed the circle, I invited the women to say the compassion phrases before going to bed at night and when they woke up in the morning. I added that even if we don't "feel" warmth and tenderness when we first begin saying the phrases, we are sowing the seeds of self-compassion, trusting that they will sprout in due time. As we would soon find out, compassion practice would help change Colleen's experience of herself and the way she could relate to Jacob.

Compassion in Our Daily Lives

The next month when the women's circle met again, Colleen was eager to tell us about something that had happened with Jacob. One evening after a particularly hard day at work, she said she'd been feeling so tired and her nerves were frayed. She was resting on the couch in the bedroom, waiting for Jacob to come home so they could make dinner together.

When she heard him open the door, she felt a surge of happiness and relief, looking forward to seeing him, to thank him for taking such good care of them—"them" now including their baby growing inside her. She listened as Jacob ran up the stairs, but when he walked into the room carrying a big paper bag, the air suddenly filled with the smell of beef burritos. Normally that would have been a welcome treat, but she was still sensitive to strong smells. Heat rose in her body along with overwhelming nausea. *How could he have done that?* She had told him that she couldn't bear the smell of burritos. *Hadn't he heard her?*

Furious, the frustration and anger poured out of her. She blamed Jacob for not caring about her, for being insensitive. She called him stupid and mean. Trying to hold down the nausea, she paced around the room, not knowing what to do with the discomfort in her body, not knowing how to calm down. Jacob tried to explain that he'd wanted to save them cooking time so they could watch a movie together after dinner, that he was sorry he forgot. Colleen couldn't hear him. As Jacob left the room, she slammed the door behind him.

Colleen paced back and forth still seething with anger. Her body was tight and her breath quick and shallow. Waves of anger kept sweeping through her. *How could he do that? Doesn't he ever listen to me? If he can't think about me, how is he going to think about a baby?* Then she sat on the bed and burst into tears. She felt a familiar ache in her chest—the pain of feeling alone, unseen, unheard. She lay down on her bed and wrapped herself in a blanket.

As Colleen closed her eyes, an image of the women in the meditation circle arose in her mind. She remembered the way they looked at her with kindness. She placed her hand on her heart and silently repeated the phrases they had learned. *I care about myself. I care about this suffering. May I open my heart to myself without fear and without judgment.* At first, she didn't feel much change but as she continued, she began to notice her heart beating slower and her breath growing deeper. *I care about myself. I forgive myself. I made a mistake, and I can try again.* Slowly the kindness of compassion was bringing Colleen back to herself.

As she lay there, she began to hear the sound of Jacob's guitar swirling up the staircase. Her heart swelled with love for her partner. *He too is suffering,* she thought. *He was trying to help and I lashed out at him again.* The words arose in her mind: *I care about your suffering, Jacob. May you be free from suffering. May I open my heart to you without fear and without judgment.* With the tenderness of compassion in her heart, Colleen got out of bed and went downstairs. When she walked into the room, Jacob looked up, a little uncertain. To his surprise, Colleen apologized for her reactivity and asked if there was anything he wanted to say to her. Feeling her genuine caring, he reached out his hand and led her to the couch. They sat down and spent the evening talking. Held by compassion, they found their way back to each other again.

When we turn toward ourselves and meet our pain with compassion, we transform the habit of self–abandonment. As we say to ourselves *Yes, this is a difficult time. Yes, I am not doing well right now. And yes, I can meet myself with love and without judgment,* we let go of pretending that everything is just fine. Acknowledging our suffering, we allow tenderness to arise. As we practice compassion for ourselves, we grow in the love and understanding of what it means to be open and kind even in the face of suffering. Carefully listening to our pain and touching it with compassion, a natural process of healing begins to unfold and we deepen in love for ourselves.

Many of us begin our journey back to ourselves with an urgent need to attend to the emotional pain and inner turmoil of self–abandonment. Turning toward our pain and holding it with the warmth of compassion is the essence of our path back to ourselves. We may first need the support of others to hold that pain, but all of us have the capacity to find the source of compassion within ourselves. Connected to the well of kindness within, we listen and respond to the cry of our heart with tenderness and understanding. As we patiently heal the wounds of the past, our heart softens, and we take ourselves back into its warm embrace.

Chapter Four

Releasing the Voice of Self–Judgment: Turning Back with Lovingkindness

After those months of healing work with Carol, I felt ready to return to IMS for the three–month retreat that coming fall. Now, after deepening in compassion, I finally felt ready to focus on lovingkindness. For the first six weeks, that would be my practice, cultivating unconditional love with the intention of opening my heart to myself and all living beings.

I started with what is traditionally taught as the first step in the practice of lovingkindness, *metta* in Pali, sending wishes of well-being to myself. I diligently repeated the phrases, *May I be happy, may I be peaceful* ... But somehow, I still couldn't open my heart to actually loving myself, and the phrases were not flowing easily. One afternoon I met again with Michele McDonald, and just as she had directed me to self-compassion during the first three-month retreat, she again offered me the clue I needed. "Lovingkindness is practiced in a gentle and easy way," she said. "The path and the goal are one and the same, this is the path of all-embracing love. So, you may want to begin your meditation in whatever way is easiest for you, maybe by sending metta to someone you already feel a warmth of love for." This instruction landed well with me. Taking the path of least resistance and allowing love to grow felt exactly like how I needed to begin.

When I went back to the hall to practice, I asked myself who would be the person my heart felt most open to. Who could I freely and wholeheartedly send thoughts of lovingkindness to? An image came to mind of the baby I was longing to have. As I sent wishes for happiness and well-being to her, I could feel the sweetness of lovingkindness arising and growing in me. In my body I felt a warm vibration, my mind was peaceful and quiet, and I felt like I had entered a chamber of love. Walking around the retreat center, I could feel that love flowing through me to others. I found myself offering metta to meditators walking down the hallways, to the person standing in front of me in the food line, to the cooks as they brought out steaming pans of food for lunch, and especially to the birds that came to the feeders. A love awakened in me that was not personal but felt larger and wider than myself. I came to understand the lines of the poet Rilke: "I live my life in widening circles / that reach out across the world." I experienced a happiness I had not known before—the happiness of an open heart.

At my next check-in with Michele, I told her how the practice was affecting me. She smiled and said now that my heart was so open to others, this would be a good time to start sending metta to myself. She suggested that I begin in the traditional way, reflecting on my beautiful qualities and wholesome deeds. "Reflecting on our own goodness," she said, "awakens lovingkindness for ourselves." Offering her own variation of the metta phrases, she guided me through each one:

May I be protected and safe from inner and outer harm.
May I be happy ... just as I am.
May I be peaceful ... with whatever is happening.
May I live my life with ease of well-being.

This version of the phrases felt deeply meaningful to me. Repeating those words over and over, wishing myself happiness and peace, I actually began holding myself with love. I let myself acknowledge some of my beautiful qualities—my courage and my love of truth. I remembered times with friends and family when I had acted out of kindness, and those moments of sending metta to others during the retreat. I began to see myself with a soft gaze, with kind eyes. I got glimpses into what it might feel like to live without judging myself harshly, without abandoning myself. As I opened to receive the lovingkindness I was sending to myself, I could feel an inner barrier dissolving and a new feeling of wholeness emerging within me. For days I was held in the joy and blessing of holding myself with a loving heart.

But these expansive experiences of lovingkindness practice can also reveal mindstates that run counter to that love. Metta is a purification practice, bringing up anything in our heart that is keeping us from loving ourselves or others. We see where our heart is not open, where we are holding onto habits of judgment, anger, or resentment. In the silence of a retreat, with nowhere to hide from our own mind, those habits can become especially apparent.

I remember one day arriving late to lunch and missing out on my favorite dish. A huge wave of anger erupted in me, and I found myself banging on the table in frustration. That was immediately followed by a barrage of judgmental thoughts. *I am a total failure at being a yogi. I can't even control my reactions.* There were also a number of times when I asked a question during the Q&A sessions in the meditation hall, and even before the teacher finished answering, I was judging myself for speaking too much, for taking up too much space, for asking stupid questions. The stark contrast between holding myself with lovingkindness and closing my heart in painful self-judgment was confusing. When I asked Michele how to work with this, she said to let those difficult feelings move through me, just observing them with mindfulness, not getting entangled in them, and when they subsided, returning to metta. That was not easy to do, but the power of my intention seemed to be working.

One morning during one of the Q&A sessions, I once again asked a question, and my mind was flooded with the voices of self-judgment berating me. My heart was racing, and I wanted to hide. Completely sunk in the pain of the judging mind, suddenly an image of Carol, my therapist, arose. I put my hand on my heart and silently recited the words she had given me when we worked together: *I care about myself.* Turning back to myself with compassion opened the way to metta, and the judgmental voices began to soften. As the phrase arose again in my mind, *May I be protected and safe from inner and outer harm,* I could feel lovingkindness giving me that protection.

When the retreat was over and I returned to "the world" again, I continued to find that when I slipped into self-judgment or anger, lovingkindness could bring me back to myself. Metta had the power to "reset" my mind and my heart and help me reconnect again with love. So, when I started leading meditation circles for women and saw that I was not alone in facing self-judgment, I knew this practice could help them transform their pain and open to loving themselves, recognizing their beauty, and knowing they deserved to be treated kindly.

Cultivating lovingkindness for ourselves, as I had learned on the retreat, is the antidote to abandoning ourselves to the voices of self-judgment. With the warm and open voice of love, we can treat ourselves as kindly as we would a close friend or a beloved family member. As we practice lovingkindness, we learn to stand by our side and unconditionally wish ourselves well in times of sorrow as well as in times of joy. As metta quiets the voice of self-judgment, we develop a loving and caring relationship with ourselves and with our world.

Getting to Know the Judging Mind

When Ilana first introduced herself to the women's circle, we could all see that she was creative and smart, and we enjoyed her playful personality. It was clear why she was a successful middle-school teacher, well-loved by her students. But as we got to know her over time, we also learned that she often struggled with a harsh inner critic.

Growing up, Ilana had been continually lectured by her father about the right way to be a woman, about how a woman should behave to get a man and keep him. "He would sit me down in his study and tell me I should be smart but not too smart," Ilana told us. "He said I should keep my hair long because men like women with long hair. He told me to not get fat. He told me very explicitly that if a man wants something from me, I should do it. He told me that men are smarter than women. Men drive better and make better decisions. He even referred to academic papers to prove his points." As an adolescent, Ilana believed that what her father was saying was true, and she even felt lucky to be getting proper training. She trusted him. And she knew that if a man found fault with her, it would be due to her own wrongdoing.

The messages Ilana received from her father settled deeply into her body, mind, and heart, and they followed her into her relationships with men. When she dated, if things didn't go well, she would hear her father's voice in her mind saying, "You're too fat, you're too opinionated, you want too much." If her date made unwanted advances, that inner voice would say, "Men and women are different biologically, you need to make more allowances for men." Starting in her late teens, Ilana got into a series of relationships with attractive, charismatic, highly intelligent—and abusive—men. She repeatedly found herself tiptoeing around them, walking on eggshells, doing everything she could to please and appease them, just as her father had conditioned her to do. Whenever she evoked their wrath, she would apologize and plead for forgiveness. Invariably, in their abusive final act, the men would leave her.

Her first husband Mark was one of these men. "Even though we have been divorced for a year and a half," Ilana told us, "his voice is still controlling how I feel about myself and the choices I make." One Sunday morning in our women's circle, what she told us made that apparent. "Last week I was all set to finally go to the annual music and dance festival here," she began. "I've wanted to go for years, and now that my *ex*–husband," she said—emphasizing the *ex*—"isn't controlling my life, I felt free to do something I love." We all laughed a little at her triumphant emphasis but quickly sobered as we saw tears rising. "His voice is still there in my mind." As we listened to her story, we could almost hear that berating voice.

"When we were married and went to parties, Mark would watch me dancing and having a good time, and then when we'd get home, he'd yell at me for hours. *You did it again. You embarrassed yourself, and me! You're always showing off, looking for attention. You make such a spectacle of yourself.* And I could hear my father's voice all over again, telling me to do what men expected, not to challenge them, to be obedient. I would get into bed and lie there thinking, *What is wrong with me? Why do I always mess things up?*

"So, when I thought about going to the festival this year," Ilana continued, "and I imagined myself joining in with everyone dancing and celebrating, that same feeling came up again. One voice inside me was saying, *Go! You'll love it!* but the other one was saying *You'll embarrass yourself. You just want attention.* And that's the voice that won. I stayed home." Having succumbed to the inner judge, Ilana spent the festival weekend feeling restless and resentful, berating herself for not honoring her own desires, wishing she was out there dancing.

As Ilana talked about how undermining those judgmental voices were for her, I noticed other women in the circle nodding in recognition, so I asked if any of them would like to share their own stories about their inner judge. Annette said the judging mind was her constant companion from the moment she opened her eyes in the morning until she went to sleep at night, even appearing in her dreams. Colleen's inner judge was persistent, argumentative, and always needed to be right. "Yes," Ilana agreed, "that judge is unforgiving and always on my case." As we continued around the circle, we could hear how that voice controlled the lives of these women in so many ways. Erin told us she could still hear the voice of the choir director in her school telling her she couldn't carry a tune, and since that moment she had never tried singing again, anywhere. In third grade, Lisa's teacher told her she was hopeless at math, and even now when she paid her bills or did her taxes, that voice kept telling her *You're not going to do this right.* Sandra told us that when she was a teenager, whenever she folded laundry, she would hear her mother's voice correcting her, and now as an adult, she couldn't do this simple task without feeling anxious, as if her mother were still looking over her shoulder telling her what she was doing wrong.

The harsh voice of the inner judge functions as the agent of self-abandonment. It creates a barrier that prevents us from experiencing our goodness. It puts us out of our hearts and distances us from love. In its presence we forget who we truly are, and we abandon our innate potential for loving and accepting ourselves. In face of that judgmental voice, we experience what Tara Brach in her book *Radical Acceptance* calls "the trance of unworthiness." As she points out, when we are lost in that trance, we see ourselves as worthless, not trustworthy, inadequate, not good enough. We dislike ourselves, speak badly about ourselves, which only deepens our loneliness, self-hatred, and self-doubt. Filled with shame, we believe that we are not worthy of love.

This judging mind holds us back from expressing ourselves fully and authentically. As we try to live within the confines of the expectations that have been imposed on us by others, we give up our power, our aliveness, and our dreams. Learning to do what is expected of us, we put aside our aspirations, telling ourselves we will get to them later or that they don't really matter. And we end up hiding or suppressing the frustration we feel at living a life that is not our own. At the mercy of the inner judge, we find ourselves trapped in habits formed in the past, reacting to life out of fear rather than responding and welcoming it with wisdom and love.

Our journey back to ourselves begins when we start to question the authority of that inner judge and the power it has over our lives. As we get to know the judging mind and its detrimental effects, out of compassion for ourselves we choose to no longer abandon ourselves but instead to turn and hold ourselves with lovingkindness.

To complete our gathering in the women's circle that day, I suggested that over the next month everyone might notice the voice of the inner judge in their daily life. "When you hear that voice in your mind telling you that something is wrong with you, pause and mentally take a step back. Not fighting or disregarding what it is saying, just see it for what it is, the voice of judgment arising from unhealed parts of your past. Let yourself be aware of that voice without falling into believing it." Standing in our closing circle, I could feel the strength of intention we all held to heal the pain of self-judgment.

Remembering Our Goodness

When we met again, the women in the circle were eager to talk about what they had learned from noticing their judgmental thoughts with mindfulness. One woman said she had become more aware of how those judgments were stopping her from doing what she wanted to do in the world. Another spoke about the relief and freedom she felt when she could see judgments as thoughts in her mind, knowing she didn't need to believe or fear them. Some spoke about the relaxation they felt in their body when their mind was not taken over by the judge.

Listening to their experiences, I realized I wanted to share with them one of my favorite poems by Galway Kinnell, "St. Francis and the Sow." As Sharon Salzberg points out in her book on lovingkindness, the poem is a beautiful way to remind us how to turn back to ourselves with love despite our self-judgments. The room was quiet as I read the poem, and I could sense how deeply they were taking it in. A few of the lines were especially meaningful for what we would be doing in our circle that day: "… sometimes it is necessary to reteach a thing its loveliness … until it flowers again from within, of self-blessing." I hoped that offering them the practice of lovingkindness would be that self-blessing for them.

"Lovingkindness, metta, is a way to open our hearts with love," I began. "Doing this practice can free us from the voice of self-judgment. Remembering that all living beings wish to be happy, in this practice we open our heart with well-wishing for ourselves and others. In the traditional way, we start by acknowledging our own beautiful qualities and our wish to be happy." Sensing a slight unease in the circle, I said, "For many of us it isn't easy to shift the habit of our mind from self-judgment to self-appreciation, so we can begin today by remembering what it feels like to be loved."

I asked them to call to mind someone who has seen their beautiful qualities, someone who appreciated and celebrated them, who did not judge them but accepted them for who they are. "Maybe you've known someone who encouraged you to begin something you'd been longing to do. Or maybe you have a relative or a close friend who treasures you. As you recall being seen and loved by them, notice how you feel in your body and in your heart." I watched as the women relaxed into this process, and soon a sense of ease appeared on many faces.

When they opened their eyes, I asked if anyone wanted to share her experience. Colleen said she had remembered the day Alison, her high school music teacher, showed up with a shining new flute and said, "This is for you." Her face glowing, Colleen told us this had been the first time someone had ever cared for her in that way. "Alison saw me. She saw my talent, and that helped me see it for myself. Receiving that flute was a turning point in my life. I feel a warmth in my heart just remembering the moment."

Erin remembered her Aunt Bess who she used to visit on summer vacations. They would do science experiments together, like testing the pH of different solutions or learning about magnetic fields. "Aunt Bess appreciated my interest in science and that gave me the confidence to go in that direction with my life. It's thanks to her that I got an engineering degree and am working to address the causes of climate change."

Annette recalled going to her Grandma Jo's house and hanging out in the kitchen with her. While her grandma baked bread or made pasta sauce from scratch, Annette would practice new dance steps she had learned that week. "Grandma Jo would stop everything she was doing and watch me dance. Her eyes sparkled. When I finished a piece, she would clap her hands with excitement and delight. Her enthusiasm helped me see that I was doing something beautiful. Her kitchen felt like an open space with endless possibility. I would fly across the floor as if it was a stage. With her I didn't need to hold myself back. I could spread my arms out and pretend to fly."

Ilana looked around at the group and said, "Well, I know that my mother loved me. I remember her stroking my hair and playing with my curls, but she never told me she was proud of me. She was a brilliant woman and was well regarded at work. At home, though, she lived in the shadow of my domineering father, and she too held herself back." Ilana took a deep breath and smiled. "During the meditation I remembered someone else. Her name was Willow. I often went to her house after school when my mom was still working. She always welcomed me with a big hug and seemed truly happy to see me. She wanted to know everything about my day, about what I had learned and what I was thinking. She would say things like 'That is a very interesting thought, tell me more.' Or 'I love your voice.' Or 'Keep writing, your poetry makes me cry.' Her words made my heart swell. I would come home feeling I had beautiful qualities in me."

Looking around at all of them, I said, "I'm moved by hearing the ways you have felt appreciated by others. Seeing our beauty and our goodness through the eyes of those who love us allows us to see it for ourselves." Now that they were in touch with the feeling of being loved and appreciated, I felt they were ready for the next part of metta practice. I suggested they get comfortable and close their eyes.

"Bringing your attention again to your body and to your heart, let yourself name some of your own beautiful qualities. Just as others saw these, you can let yourself recognize them. You might acknowledge your creativity or your truthfulness, maybe your kindness or your patience, your adventurous spirit or your courage in exploring your inner life. As you notice these qualities, allow yourself to rejoice in the gifts you bring to the world."

After a few minutes, we opened up the circle again for sharing. Ilana told us she appreciated her love of beauty, the way she sees color and patterns in the trees when she walks in the woods. Colleen said she appreciated her fierce courage that allowed her to speak up and fight for justice. Erin was happy that she was doing something to make a difference for the planet. And Annette rejoiced in preparing herself hearty salads from greens she grew in her backyard. The room was filled with a sense of joy and appreciation. It was as if the whole group had grown taller and more confident, as if each of them was able to more fully take her place in the circle.

Reflecting on our goodness reconditions our mind, creating a new habit to replace the negative condemning voice of the judge. As we focus on our wholesome qualities, the voice of judgment begins to soften, and we get a glimpse into the experience of self-love. We begin to discover the part of ourselves that is happy to be alive, the part of ourselves that greets each day with curiosity and enthusiasm, the part of us that feels and expresses joy.

As we acknowledge and delight in our innate goodness, we discover that we are not the person our inner judge has been telling us we are. We see ourselves in a new light. While we don't ignore or deny areas of our lives where we can grow, we find that there is already much to celebrate and rejoice in. With that sense of appreciation, we develop the courage to be ourselves and to enter the upward spiral of turning back to ourselves with lovingkindness.

> ## Seeing Ourselves with Kind Eyes
>
> ~
>
> Bring to mind someone who cares about you. It may be a friend, a family member, a teacher, or even a pet. Imagine them standing a few feet in front of you and looking at you with kind eyes. With or without words, they are telling you how happy they are to see you, how much they appreciate you for who you are. Bring your attention to your body and notice what it feels like to take in that love. You may feel a warming in your heart, perhaps a smile on your face. Let your attention rest on these feelings for a few moments, and then set the intention to carry this feeling of being loved into the rest of your day.
>
> (Inspired by an exercise offered by Dr. Diane Poole Heller)

After a short break for a stretch, we all returned to the circle. "Now that we have begun to open our hearts to ourselves by seeing our goodness, we are ready to take the next step in lovingkindness practice, which is sending thoughts of well-wishing to ourselves and then extending those wishes to others." I explained that by repeating the metta phrases, we were sowing seeds of love, creating the conditions for love to sprout in our hearts. "As you repeat these phrases inviting happiness and well-being, you might imagine a meadow where the seeds of wildflowers are being blown by the wind and gently landing on the ground, trusting that the rain will come, that the soil will provide, and the flowers will bloom."

With metta in my own heart, I slowly offered them the phrases I had learned from Michele my meditation teacher.

When the meditation was over, I could feel the palpable shift in the room, as if together in the warmth of connection, we had all been touched by the sacred. In a calm and steady voice, Ilana told us that the phrase she found especially meaningful was "May I be happy, just as I am." It reminded her that she was not "too much," that her exuberance was a gift, not something to hold back or be ashamed of. "I've finally found the practice I was looking for," she said. "I feel like this can unfurl those buds of self-love that were mentioned in the poem."

Annette told us that the phrases brought up the feeling she felt when she was out in her garden, connected to the earth and to the plants. She said the process made her feel grateful to be alive. For a few minutes, the voice of the judge had been completely silent, and she had felt a deep sense of belonging and of being at home in herself.

Colleen added that the metta phrases felt like a loving voice she had rarely heard before. "They sounded warm and kind, like something a mother would say to a child. It felt like a balm to my heart." She was articulating what many of us were feeling that day. The practice of metta was offering her the love she had been longing for since she was very young, and she could now offer it to herself from the depths of her own heart.

As the circle was ending, I suggested that as a daily practice they continue sending themselves love and affirming their beautiful qualities. Ilana summed it all up by pointing out how metta was bringing healing to what we had all been struggling with: "As I send love to myself, I feel like that voice of the judge is getting softer."

The Pain of Seeking Perfection

While it is possible to soften the voice of the inner judge by shifting our attention to our wholesome qualities, sometimes the voice of judgment can be so overwhelming that even mindful attention doesn't help us relieve its impact. When we find ourselves lost in such a painful mindstate, we may need to first heal the wounds of our past before we can turn back to ourselves with love and appreciation. That healing is what would allow Laura to turn back and hold herself in lovingkindness.

When Laura arrived for her first appointment with me, she sat down on the edge of the couch, looking as if she was trying not to take up too much space. She had barely started talking when her eyes filled with tears. "I'm thinking of dropping out of art school," she said quietly, gazing at the floor. "No matter how hard I try, I'm just not good enough." She looked up and, choking back tears, said, "I feel like an utter failure."

Laura told me she was a student of fine arts at a well-known university a couple of hours away. She had aspired to use her art for social change, especially to portray the injustice evident in the poverty she observed on her walk to campus every day. But with both passion and frustration in her voice, she said she had to make sure her art was good, "really good … otherwise, why would it matter? What value would it have?" So, she spent countless hours revising her work, tearing up her drawings and starting again, doing them over and over until she was satisfied … sort of.

Laura had first heard the word "perfect" when she was four or five years old. "I remember sitting at the kitchen table, drawing a flower. I loved my flower. It had pink petals and an orange center. I was proud of myself. I called my mother to see what I had made, but somehow she wasn't happy with it. She started correcting me—something she did a lot—making me draw the flower again. After I'd tried five or six times, she finally said: 'This is perfect!' She kissed me and told me she loved me and what a good artist I was. But it wasn't my flower any longer. It had become her flower."

Laura learned that she was worthy of love—not for simply being alive or for doing things her own way—but only when she met her mother's standards and expectations. That voice demanding perfection had found its place inside her as her inner judge.

Kristin Neff, author of *Self-Compassion: The Proven Power of Being Kind to Yourself*, points out that, as children, many of us receive the message that it is not enough for us to simply participate in our lives and be happy. Neff writes: "Our competitive culture tells us we need to be special and above average to feel good about ourselves, but we can't all be above average at the same time. There is always someone richer, more attractive, or successful than we are… . Our sense of self-worth bounces around like a ping-pong ball, rising and falling in lock-step with our latest success or failure."

Like that bouncing ping-pong ball, Laura's experience of her self-worth had fallen or risen as a child, depending on the regard of her parents. By the time she was in high school, her parents were telling her that she had great potential as an artist, that she was "exceptional," and that someday she could be showing her art in a prominent gallery in Manhattan. When she won prizes and they were happy, she felt good about herself. But when her work in a competition was overlooked, she felt despondent, knowing how disappointed they were, and she'd often stay in bed for several days, depressed, overcome by shame, not wanting to see or be seen by anyone.

After graduating from high school and enrolling in a prestigious art program, Laura found that she was one of many talented young artists, and not being singled out for accolades left her feeling lost. During the weekly work reviews, she nervously awaited comments from her teachers and peers. Inside her, the judgmental voices would be questioning: *Am I good enough to be here? Do they like my work? Do they like me?* At the slightest hint of criticism from her teachers or suggestions for improvement, she would feel as if those inner voices were crushing her. She often left the critiques filled with self-judgment, doubting her talent, thinking she would never make it as an artist, wondering what to do with her life. Those judgmental thoughts carried her into the downward spiral of self-abandonment.

Brené Brown, social scientist and author, says the "pursuit of perfection" is one of the ways we avoid feeling shame. When our sense of self-worth has been damaged through negative judgments or through failing in face of high expectations from others, we can find that we are exhausting ourselves by trying to achieve more, by trying to prove that we have value. In the pursuit of perfection, we abandon ourselves, pushing beyond our limits. We ignore the messages of our bodies and our hearts, begging us to slow down, asking us to think again about what we're really after.

Like Laura, many of us are led by the harsh voice of the inner judge into a downward spiral of shame and self-doubt. Fearing that if we are seen as failing or needy, we will not be loved or we will be abandoned, we hide our feelings of unworthiness and insecurity from others and even from ourselves. It can take an emotional breakdown, a loss, a physical illness, or an episode of depression to reveal these tender feelings, asking us to at last honor our authentic and vulnerable self. In such times of crisis, we finally realize that the high standards we had been pursuing cannot give us the love and happiness we are longing for, nor do they pacify the voice of the inner judge.

By the time she came to see me, Laura had realized that the goal she was pushing toward was not supporting her aspirations as an artist. She hid her feelings from her classmates and friends, holding up the front of a strong, capable woman ... until one day the facade fell. After a particularly hard day at the studio, she arrived home late at night and burst into tears. Her mind was overcome by the negative thoughts she had been harboring for months. *This isn't working. I'm failing. I will never make it.* With her heart beating so hard she thought it would break, and unable to stop the sobs wracking her body, Laura made a phone call to a friend who lovingly suggested she seek help. Laura's willingness to show up at my office was the first step on her journey back to herself.

Healing the Pain of the Judging Mind

After coming for a couple of sessions, Laura decided to drop one of her classes and lighten up her schedule for a while. It seemed to be helping, but one afternoon she arrived at my office feeling disheartened again. "That harsh voice of the judge is not budging," she said. "I know it quite well by now, but I just can't get it to go away. All these thoughts keep going through my mind—that I can't get things right, that something's wrong with me."

"It sounds like that judge doesn't take any breaks, Laura. When you hear it, do you have a sense of whose voice that might be?"

After a moment Laura said, "It must be my mother's. It has the same feeling as when she made me draw the flower over and over. I've been thinking about this a lot since starting to see you. She never had a chance to go to college. In fact, she wanted to go to art school, but her parents couldn't afford it. After high school she had to get a job. And then when I came along, she definitely didn't have any time for art. I can see now that she wanted me to have what she didn't have, and she was afraid that if I didn't get it right, I would fail and end up like her."

Laura took a deep breath and sat back. "So, of course I am staying up till midnight, redoing my paintings multiple times. That fear I picked up from my mother is still in me. Whenever I stand in front of my peers and my teachers for a review, I am waiting and hoping for my mother to say, 'This is perfect.'"

When we turn toward the inner judge and listen carefully, we often discover that underlying the harsh, undermining, and condescending voice is fear. It may be the fear that one of our parents felt, or the fear felt by a teacher or someone earlier in our lives who was trying to protect us from failure, embarrassment, or hurt. But caught up in their own fears, not trusting us to do the "right thing," they corrected us, scolded us until we finally did what they wanted, what they thought would keep us safe. Laura was beginning to understand that her real struggle was not so much about getting the approval of her teachers and peers but rather about knowing who she could be without that drive to perfection that started when she was a child. That realization would open her up to begin learning how to love herself.

"That is a powerful insight, Laura," I said kindly. "Can you let yourself close your eyes now and remember that voice criticizing you, saying you're not good enough, that you're not doing it right? How do you feel in your body when you hear that?"

"I feel a lump in my throat," she said softly, and touching her chest, she added, "and I feel a pain in my heart, right here."

"Let's stay with those sensations for a few moments. You can leave your hand there, over your heart, meeting that painful feeling with kindness."

As Laura gently patted her chest, a small stream of tears rolled down her cheeks. Meeting the sensations with tenderness and care was opening her to emotions that had been held in her body for years.

"As you breathe into those sensations and hold them gently, can you tell me how old you are when you're feeling this? Does it bring up a memory of a place or a time?"

"I feel like I'm very young, four or five years old. I can see myself sitting at the kitchen table that day I drew the flower."

"Now, as that young Laura, what emotions are you feeling?"

"Frustrated," she answered. "Discouraged, confused. I don't know if I am good or bad. I don't understand why my mother keeps asking me to draw the flower again. And I am scared of making mistakes. I don't want to disappoint her again." Laura's face was flushed, and she clenched her fists as she spoke.

"Still being young Laura, what would you like to hear from your mother?"

After a moment she said softly, "I want to hear that the flower I drew the first time was beautiful. I want my mother to recognize that I am good just as I am. I want her to love what I am doing. I want her to love me."

"And if you could be that loving mother, what would you say to young Laura now?"

Laura's face softened as she spoke. "Take your time, little one, there is no right or wrong way to draw a flower. Your flower is beautiful."

"And how does that make young Laura feel?"

Laura smiled. "I can see it makes her happy. She's smiling too."

I waited, knowing this was a turning point for Laura. When she opened her eyes, she said, "When we started, my chest felt really tight, but now the edges are softening and opening. And the lump in my throat is almost gone." I could see how relaxed her body looked. She looked at me and said, "I think that little girl can feel good about herself now." Smiling, Laura poured herself a glass of water and slowly drank it.

"Now that young Laura is feeling heard, let's bring ourselves back to that inner judge. How is she feeling right now?"

"I see her differently now. My inner judge, just like my mother, has been afraid for me. She worries about me and doesn't trust me to finish art school. So, she keeps insisting that I work harder. She doesn't want me to fail."

"Are you afraid too? Are you afraid that you might fail?" I asked Laura tenderly. And as if a dam had broken open, she burst into tears, the fear of failure underlying the judgmental voice pouring out of her.

I waited until the wave of grief and fear subsided. Wiping her eyes, Laura said, "I was never able to let myself feel those deep feelings, but they were always there, like an undercurrent of tension in my body." She took a deep breath. "I feel lighter and like I can breathe more freely. And I see something more clearly now—I'm not a child any longer. I am twenty-four years old and actually quite capable." As she uttered those words, Laura's posture changed, and a look of confidence came over her face. She smiled and sighed. "Maybe I don't need to do each painting over and over endlessly. If I like what I've done, maybe at some point I can just trust that it is good."

When Laura returned to my office a couple of weeks later, it was obvious that something had softened in her. "I've been feeling a little more relaxed," she said. "At least I wasn't fighting with myself all the time."

Knowing Laura was ready to build a new relationship with herself, I introduced her to lovingkindness practice. Recognizing her tendency to strive for perfection, I emphasized that this is a gentle practice and that change happens gradually over time. "As one of my meditation teachers, Sharon Salzberg, says, our mind will get filled with lovingkindness moment by moment, just as a bucket gets filled with water, drop by drop. Each time we recite the phrases, we are adding drops to the bucket, filling our hearts with lovingkindness." After we had spent some time with each of the phrases, I asked what the experience had been like for her.

"With the words 'May I be protected and safe,' my body felt warm and my shoulders dropped," she said. "Something in me heard that I don't have to hurt myself with all those negative judgments and by pushing so hard." She took a breath. "And 'May I be happy just as I am' felt like a totally new idea to me. I feel like my life has been only about achieving and producing in order to make other people happy, never about me being happy. And what does happiness even mean to me? Trying to be perfect is not it, so maybe it's more about softening the voice of the judge and being kinder to myself."

Laura's face lit up. "That next phrase, 'being peaceful with whatever is happening,' feels like taking back my power. It's about not getting so upset by those reviews. In the art world, I know that sometimes I'll be praised and other times I'll be criticized, and for sure feelings will come up—and I also know I will be okay. That for me is the message of that phrase. And in the last one, 'May I live with ease,' the word *ease* sounds lovely. It feels light. I know that striving and getting attached to results is working against me, and I am most creative when my mind is relaxed." She smiled. "So yes, may I live with ease."

Opening Our Heart in Widening Circles

When the women's circle met again, Ilana told us that sending lovingkindness to herself during the past few weeks had been like turning on the "love channel" to replace the "judging channel" in her mind. She said that after ten or fifteen minutes of reciting the metta phrases, a feeling of warmth and safety would come over her, and a kind and loving voice would replace the harsh voice of the judge in her mind.

After each of the women had talked about the effect of holding themselves with lovingkindness, I introduced the final step in the practice, sending metta out in growing circles until we open our heart to all living beings. "The nature of lovingkindness is boundless," I began. "Its source has no limits, and it can continue to flow endlessly. This beautiful quality of lovingkindness reminds me of a story. In my early twenties, I went on a long hike with a small group of friends through the red granite mountain range called Farsh–Abu–Hsheib in the Sinai Desert. After a couple of challenging days backpacking and carrying water on our backs, we came upon a small oasis where water was flowing in a series of small cascading pools. When one pool was full to the brim, the water flowed down to the next. Metta is like that. Like water flowing from one cascading pool into another, when our heart is full of love for ourselves, that warmth flows from us to others. And just as that pool in Sinai was flowing for anyone, metta can flow from us not only to those we love but to people we don't know and even to those we may struggle to love."

Anchored again in lovingkindness for ourselves, we began expanding our wishes for the happiness and well-being of others. I invited them to call to mind someone they felt grateful to. "Traditionally, in metta practice this is called a 'benefactor,' someone who has brought good into our lives, someone we hold in high regard. Sending metta to this person opens our heart even more."

I guided them to next think of someone they felt close to, "a dear friend," someone who brings a smile to their face. We then went on to send wishes for well-being to someone we might see from time to time but may never even speak with. This "neutral person," as they are referred to in the practice, might be someone we pass in the park when we're walking or someone we sometimes see at the grocery store, and we remember that they too wish to be happy.

And then I introduced them to a challenging category, sending metta to someone who is a "difficult person" for us. This might be someone we are in conflict with or have been hurt by. Even if our heart has not yet opened to them, by saying the phrases with intention, we begin to soften the barrier that seems to separate us. Extending well-wishing to this person does not necessarily mean that we have to develop a close relationship with them, but it allows us to open our heart enough to genuinely wish them freedom from suffering.

As I introduced the final step in the practice, *May all beings everywhere be happy,* I was brought back to my experience on the three-month retreat of feeling a fully opened heart, and I delighted in inviting all these women into knowing that joy. We ended the session by bringing our attention back to ourselves, appreciating our courage and our willingness to open our heart so wide.

After the meditation Ilana told us that at first her "love channel" had opened to her students, especially those who needed some extra love and care. Then a memory had come up of her mother stroking her curls. "I could almost feel the softness of her fingers in my hair. She felt so close, as if we were sitting here together." She told us that when she sent the phrases to her mother, it felt like her heart was overflowing with gratitude. But her father was in the category of the difficult person. As she reminded herself that he too wished to be happy, something in her began to soften, and she was able to send even him wishes for ease and well-being. "What a relief it was to not be angry at him for a few minutes," she said.

Annette told us that she had started sending metta to the plants in her garden. "It was easy to feel lovingkindness for the tomato plants. They're growing so tall, and the fruit on the vines is turning red, almost ready to be harvested." But when it came to some of the bugs, it got harder. "When I imagined the caterpillars and beetles eating my kale, I had to pause," she said laughing. "I just wanted them out! *It's my kale. It's my garden. Get out of here!* In order to stop being so mad at them, I had to think about their beautiful colors and their matter-of-fact way of roaming around my garden. I reminded myself that they were just living their lives, like me, eating what they needed to survive. I then imagined removing them one by one and putting them in a meadow. When they were out of my garden, not devouring my plants, I could truly wish them to be happy." We all joined her in laughter.

When we practice sending lovingkindness to all living beings, we go beyond the limits of caring only for those we already know or love. We open our hearts to the multitude of life forms, sending metta to all beings everywhere. As we do that, we are letting go of the judging mind and sincerely, unconditionally, wishing happiness for all. When we experience lovingkindness as boundless, we know that our heart, in the words of Sharon Salzberg, is as wide as the world.

The Courage to Be Ourselves

Reflecting on my own journey, I can see that my tendency to judge myself has diminished over the years, but it is not totally gone. At times I am still hard on myself when I think I have made a mistake. I might feel anxiety in the pit of my stomach, or my heart starts racing after doing or saying what I think is the wrong thing, like the time I put a dent in the car or when I have hurt Ian's feelings by criticizing him. But as I have learned to bring awareness and compassion to those experiences, something significant has changed. Instead of spiraling down into self-abandonment, I can hear the voice of the inner judge more as a "mindfulness bell." It wakes me up to the pain I am in and is my cue to turn back to myself with lovingkindness.

Abiding in lovingkindness changes our relationship to ourselves and to the world around us. The boundaries we feel between us and "the other" begin to shift. We feel less alone, less alienated, and less lonely. We become more loving not only in our hearts but also in our actions.

As Ilana deepened in lovingkindness, softening the judgmental voice inside her, she grew to trust herself as a vibrant, exuberant woman free to express herself fully. For the first time since her childhood, she danced without the voice of the judge haunting her. She joined a free-form dance class where she could let her body move and sway the way it wanted to. And the next summer, when the music and dance festival was held again, she didn't hold herself back. Knowing there is room in this world for all of who she is, she went out there dancing.

As Laura continued to hold herself with lovingkindness, she became more daring and willing to take risks in her artwork, feeling less restricted by what others might say or think. As she relaxed into her own unique life as an artist, the habit of judging herself by someone else's standards fell away, and her intention to use art for social change reawakened. She began offering art classes in elementary schools and delighted in how enthusiastic second and third graders could be about their own work. One day in the classroom, she sat down at one of the tables, took a piece of paper and some oil pastels, and drew her flower again. There it was, pink petals and an orange center. She smiled, sending thoughts of lovingkindness to both her young and adult selves, no longer abandoning either one.

Practicing metta reminds us of our own innate goodness, affirming that we are deserving of love. Growing in lovingkindness, we discover our capacity to accept ourselves, and we can relax into being who we are, as Pema Chodron puts it, "fundamentally open-minded, open-hearted, worthy, and good." Holding ourselves with love and listening to our wise and compassionate self, we embrace our strengths and our vulnerabilities. Our inherent beauty, aliveness, creativity, and joy naturally awaken. No longer held back by the voice of self-judgment, we abide in our heart, holding ourselves and all beings with lovingkindness.

CHAPTER FIVE

Coming Home to Our Bodies: Turning Back to Joy and Aliveness

※

Our bodies are the sacred vehicles through which we live and know the world. The life force moves through us as our breath, our movement, and our energy. Our senses open us to seeing, hearing, smelling, tasting, and touching. Alive in our bodies, we know where we are, what we are doing, and what we are feeling. With our bodies we dance, run, swim, and play. They are our instrument for creating art, music, gardens, books, and computer programs. For many of us, they are the way we bring life into the world. Through our voice, touch, facial expression, posture, and movement, we communicate love, intimacy, connection—and also anxiety, frustration, rage, disapproval, or rejection. Our bodies let us know when our basic needs for nourishment, safety, connection, and rest are satisfied, and conversely, when we are depleted and need to take care of ourselves.

When we consider the amazing gifts and power of our bodies, the intricate ways they work, the ways they serve us, and the capacity they have to heal from injury and ailment, we might expect to feel only gratitude and appreciation toward them. And yet many of us feel conflicted and ambivalent about our body. At times we may feel the exhilaration and ecstasy of being in a physical body, but at other times living in our body may bring up feelings of fear, anger, guilt, or shame. When we judge our body as somehow wrong, speak badly about it, or forget to care for it, we are abandoning ourselves.

We might stand in front of mirrors, scrutinizing the size and shape of our belly, our hips, and our breasts. We might judge ourselves harshly for the color and shade of our skin or the texture and style of our hair. We might examine our face for pimples and blemishes after watching TV commercials advertising a new line of skin products. We might end up abandoning our body for the sake of cultural ideas of what an ideal woman should look like.

Some of us judge ourselves for not being strong enough, not capable enough, not athletic enough. Maybe we were the girls who stood on the sidelines at school sports events, not being chosen for a team, and so we still choose now to opt out of a family frisbee game. Or maybe we feel a tug in our heart when we see a woman jogging in tight leggings and colorful running shoes, thinking *I could never do that. I am not one of those women.*

We may struggle with our bodies when we are contending with persistent pain, prolonged illness, or an unexpected accident. We may feel pulled down by the invisible pain of fibromyalgia, fear a return of breast cancer, or get angry at our body when chronic fatigue prevents us from completing simple daily chores. In the face of sickness or disability, we may feel let down by our bodies, helpless, or hopeless, separate and different from others, fearing that no one really understands what we feel.

Some of us have looked to our body for the fulfillment of birthing a child but instead faced infertility, miscarriages, or stillbirths. We may have chosen to have an abortion and yet find ourselves struggling with guilt and sadness for that loss. Some of us choose not to have children but may contend with the disappointment of our parents or grandparents for not meeting family expectations. Whatever the reason for not taking on the role of motherhood, we may find ourselves questioning our value and wholeness as women.

Some of us feel confused, conflicted, and disconnected from our sexual energy. We may judge ourselves for not feeling sexually "attractive," not having a strong enough sex drive, or not being able to sexually please our partner. Or we may feel sexually alive but compelled to harness our passion, concerned that we might be seen as "promiscuous" or "oversexed."

Some of us, drawn to romantic and sexual relationships outside of the heterosexual norm, hold back, afraid of flouting cultural standards that say sex should occur only between women and men. We might be afraid of coming out as lesbian, bisexual, pansexual, or asexual. We may identify as gender nonconforming and feel uncomfortable in our bodies, not at home with the gender we were assigned at birth. Those of us who identify as part of the LGBTQ+ community may struggle to be treated equally and even to get respectful health care.

Some of us have suffered sexual or physical abuse. This may have happened to us by family members or family friends when we were children, and we were told to remain silent. We may have been assaulted on a college campus, in the military, in a hospital, in a healthcare clinic, or in our own home. In order to survive, or afraid of not being believed, we may have stayed silent or disconnected from our bodies, and now are left feeling desecrated, anxious, depressed, shut down.

In our culture many of us lose our love for our body as we age. We may look at ourselves in the mirror and see only the wrinkles, gray hair, sagging skin, and untoned muscles of an older woman we don't recognize and might not like. And although we may still feel physically strong, and sexually alive, in the world around us we may feel invisible, unattractive, of little value. We may notice that our body and mind are actually slowing down. We may need more rest and don't remember things as well as we used to. We may feel confused or betrayed by our body.

At any age, some of us abandon ourselves by not caring for our body. Maybe we don't eat well, don't get enough sleep or exercise, or don't have regular health checkups. Maybe we feel we don't deserve to take care of our body and then feel so much shame about ways we have neglected ourselves that we continue in the same unhealthy patterns. Not caring for our body might be the result of challenging circumstances. Many of us don't have the money to afford good food or health insurance. We may be single mothers or sole providers in a household, working long hours at a job or multiple jobs and then continuing to work when we get home, taking care of children or elderly parents. In our stressed culture, many of us literally do not have the time or the energy to exercise or nurture ourselves adequately.

In all these ways we may lose a close, intimate, and loving connection with our body. We may forget that it is a sacred part of our whole being, not separate from our mind and heart. Distant from or ashamed of our body, we may feel separate from life. No matter why or how we find ourselves here, when we notice we have abandoned our body, we can always turn back with kindness and begin to find our way home to ourselves. As we reinhabit our body, we awaken to experience life more fully, and we open to the joy of living in our one precious home.

Returning to Our Body

Janet was in her early thirties when she first came to see me for counseling. She was tired of feeling heavy and unattractive, and her knees had started hurting. Through her twenties she had tried various diets and enrolled in exercise classes. Her weight had gone up and down somewhat, but she'd finally given up. "Most of the time I just wish I didn't have a body," she said. "And I hate the idea of lugging it around for the rest of my life. Especially this big flabby belly. But the worse I feel, the more I eat. I don't like my body, and I sure can't imagine finding anyone who would ... you know, like a partner or lover or something."

I asked Janet to tell me if there had been a time when she did feel comfortable in her body. "When I was a little girl," she said, "I loved being in my body. It was fun and easy. I was always outside jumping rope, playing T–ball, riding my bike. I had no sense of there being anything wrong with me. I didn't even think about my body. I was just in it. And then when I was about ten years old, everything changed. Weight loss programs were popular in our town, and my mom was really into them. Women used to go there to socialize, talk about their diets, and weigh themselves. Every weekend she would pile us all into the car and take us to one of her programs. I hated those places and cringed every time she said, "Time to go!" I always looked for an excuse to stay home. I was happy with my body as it was. I didn't feel overweight. But my mother was determined, and according to her charts, we were all too heavy. I guess getting us to those programs was her way to take care of us."

The messages Janet had received from her mother were fraught with judgment and attachment to the idea of the "right kind of body," thin and well–toned. By the time she was in high school, it was clear to her that she did not have the "ideal body" everyone seemed to want. Sitting at the lunch table in the school cafeteria, she listened to girls talking about their weight, getting praise for losing a pound, complaining bitterly about gaining one. The boys paid attention to those slim, athletic looking girls, and she was ignored. She began avoiding looking at herself in mirrors, hiding behind oversized clothing, and doing whatever she could to distance herself from her body. Janet, who had so loved being fully alive as a young girl, now found herself in a downward spiral of self–abandonment.

Janet is not alone in her struggle against our cultural standards. Until very recently the only body type featured by models and glamorous movie stars was *thin*, sometimes too thin, and media and advertising capitalized on that image. The social impact was revealed in a major research project released in 2015: 80 percent of seventeen–year–old girls in the United States were unhappy with their body, and 80 percent of teenage girls feared gaining weight and being in a large body.[1]

When self-esteem gets equated with one body type, everyone else is left feeling that something is wrong with them. Even though metabolism or genetic inheritance might cause some women's bodies to naturally carry more weight—or less weight—than average, many continue to measure themselves against those societal norms and judge themselves when they fail to fit into them.

These concerns about body weight can develop into an unhealthy relationship to food and eating. Some women develop what is known as "disordered eating." They may skip a meal or compulsively overeat or have stringent rituals around food. They may have candy or chips stashed away in their drawers and closets and eat them only in hiding. They may get caught in a "diet cycle," joining a certain plan, restricting the kinds and amounts of food they eat for several weeks and then, in a moment of stress, break their self-imposed rules, overeat, and the cycle begins all over again. Some develop a diagnosable "eating disorder," a mental health condition that can be severe and persistent and can even manifest as a dangerous rejection of the body. Being caught in any of these habits and cycles may leave a woman in despair, hating her body and not trusting her ability to be healthy, which only perpetuates the cycle.

- Only approximately half of those with eating disorders seek help.[2]

- 10,200 deaths each year in the United States are directly a result of eating disorders—this is one death every 52 minutes.[3]

- About 26 percent of people with eating disorders attempt suicide.[4]

Hating or rejecting our body sometimes means that we hate or reject all of who we are. For Janet, turning back to herself would mean not only learning how to connect with her body again but also learning how to love herself. The two would go hand in hand.

When Janet finished telling her story, she looked at me with a troubled expression. "Where do we go from here?" she asked, almost in tears. "I feel trapped."

I assured her that there was a way to turn back to her body and live in it again with comfort and ease. "It might take some time," I said, "but we can find ways to begin."

"Let's start with you telling me a little more about your relationship to your body. What is that like for you day to day?"

Janet paused and then looking down, she said softly, "There's an ongoing stream of judgments that starts when I get dressed in the morning, usually with some harsh language. Then I stand there in the kitchen fighting with myself about what to eat and what not to eat. I often just end up grabbing a doughnut on the way to work. I feel so ashamed of how I look that I don't even go for walks." Janet glanced nervously around the room and turned back to me. "I don't really have a relationship with my body."

I could sense the deep sadness behind that statement. "Janet," I said, "it sounds like every time you are aware of your body, it feels like a struggle. It must be very hard to live this way." Her eyes filled with tears, and we sat together quietly as the pain she had been keeping to herself released. I recognized in Janet's face the sense of relief that can come from being understood and seen in a caring way. When she was ready, I asked if we could try a short mindfulness meditation as a way for her to experience being in her body without judgment, just being present to what she was feeling and perceiving in the moment.

Turning to our body with mindfulness is a way we can begin to repair the sense of separation and distance we may feel. Paying attention to the body without judgment and with kindness, we start forming a new relationship with it. We learn to be present for both pleasant and unpleasant sensations, and we strengthen our ability to stay connected to our body and appreciate it even in the face of discomfort, physical pain, or illness. I knew that beginning to inhabit her body by being present with what she was experiencing could eventually lead Janet back to loving herself.

Janet looked a little doubtful. "Being present without judging myself seems almost impossible, but I'll try," she said.

Knowing how hard it might be for Janet to feel connected to her body after years of avoiding it, I wanted to make sure we would start in a gentle way. "You can begin by closing your eyes and noticing the feeling of your body sitting on the couch, your back against the pillows, your thighs touching the cushions." I waited as she settled into her body and then continued. "With kindness and caring attention, let yourself feel the sensation of your hands resting in your lap … and the feeling of your feet touching the floor. You can bring your attention to the movement of your breath and notice how your chest and abdomen expand with the inhalation and contract with the exhalation. Stay in touch with what your body is experiencing."

After guiding her in this way for a few minutes, I paused. When Janet opened her eyes, she said, "It wasn't easy to stay with my breath, but your voice brought me back when my mind wandered. By the time you finished, I felt like I started getting a sense of my body once in a while."

I appreciated Janet for being willing to be mindful of her body, and then suggested another mindfulness process to bring her into touch with her present experience. "What else do you notice right in this moment with your senses, Janet?" I asked. "You might look out the window and see trees, sky, clouds. Just noticing. Just seeing. Or feel the temperature of the air on your skin. Just feeling." A smile appeared on Janet's face as she gazed out the window for a few moments. When she turned back to me, she looked a little more relaxed. She stretched her arms over her head and said, "That was really moving, just letting myself pause and take in what I see. I even noticed my breath a few times. It has been years since I appreciated anything my body could do."

"You can use this basic mindfulness practice to turn back to your body at any time, Janet," I said. "For instance, when you leave the room today, you might notice the coolness when your hand touches the doorknob. Walking outside, you might feel the sensation of the wind blowing through your hair and the warmth of the sun on your skin. When you get home, you might notice the scent of the flowers in your garden. And tonight, when you put your head on the pillow, let yourself feel your whole body relaxing and being held by the bed."

Janet was listening carefully. "But it's not always nice and pleasant to be in my body."

"Yes, I understand. When that happens, try to be present with those sensations too, in a gentle, kind, and caring way."

"I like the idea of being gentler with myself. That might help me stop hating my body so much," Janet said.

Being present in our body with moment–by–moment attention can be a rich and enlivening experience, one that some of us might not have felt since we were young girls. But it can also bring us in touch with feelings we have been trying to avoid for years. Finding a simple activity that we like and engaging in it mindfully can be the key to beginning a new relationship with our body. I wanted to offer this possibility to Janet.

"Let's think of something you enjoy doing that you could practice with mindfulness this coming week. Do you like to garden, play an instrument, dance, cook?" I suggested.

Janet leaned forward and eagerly said, "I love to bake bread. It's one of my favorite things to do. I could do that."

"I love it. You can take the whole bread baking process as your meditation. Feel your arms as you reach for the bag of flour. Notice the smell of the yeast. Bring your attention to your hands as you knead the dough." By the time the session was over, Janet was looking forward to practicing being present in her body rather than wishing she could ignore or escape it.

As we turn to our body with curiosity and kindness, we begin to befriend it and create a caring relationship with it. By paying mindful attention to what she was experiencing as she baked bread, Janet would start to discover the aliveness that she had been missing for so long.

When she arrived for our next session, she immediately began telling me what had happened. "That exercise you suggested took me back to my childhood. I used to bake with my grandma, and doing this reminded me of that feeling I had as a child, of being in my body without any worries."

"That is beautiful," I said. "Can you tell me what you noticed as you were baking?"

"The first thing I paid attention to was the feeling of the glass jar with the flour. It was cool and smooth, and I could feel the slightly raised brand name on the side. I noticed the sticky feeling of the wet batter on my fingers as I mixed the flour and water and yeast in the bowl. I didn't like that part so much, but as I added more flour, the dough began to feel soft and warm. Then I loved the feeling of forming the loaves, and I especially liked punching them down after they had time to rise. When the bread was in the oven, the house filled with a heavenly smell. And, of course, the biggest reward was the taste. That was the best 'homework' you could have given me."

I smiled, grateful that Janet was ready to reconnect with her body in a positive way. "Now that you have had such a rewarding experience of being mindful of your body while baking, you might try expanding the practice. When you're preparing a meal, for example, let yourself slow down. Pay attention to the sensations in your hands as you chop and stir the food, to the aromas filling the kitchen, to the colors and shapes of the food you are preparing. Before you sit down to eat, pause again. You might want to appreciate your efforts and allow a moment of thankfulness for the food you are about to enjoy. As you take the first bites, take joy in the pleasure of eating, slowly taking in the smells, the tastes, and the textures of the food. Feel yourself being nurtured by it all. Listen to your body. Notice when you feel satisfied, and as you put down your utensils, thank yourself for caring for yourself in this way."

"Learning to eat mindfully has been a journey," Janet said when we met a few weeks later. "Sometimes I remember to be present and at other times I forget. There were days when the cravings got the best of me and I couldn't stop eating, even when I was no longer hungry. But I noticed that when I managed to pay attention and slow it all down, I felt better about myself. And I even started making some healthier choices in what I am eating, not because I am trying to change the way I look—not like my mother's diet routine—but rather to change the way I feel in my body. All of this seems to be helping change the way I feel about myself. This new 'me' might not be much smaller than the old me, but she already feels a little happier." As Janet continued these mindfulness practices, the painful habits of judgment would begin to diminish, allowing her to come home to her body and care for it with kindness. And she would begin recovering some of the joy she knew as a young girl living in her body.

Remembering Our Aliveness

Let yourself recall a time when you felt fully alive in your body. Maybe it was when you were a child playing games outside, or maybe more recently when you were dancing or out walking or playing a sport. What did you feel in your body and in your heart at that time? Notice how your senses were alive in that experience. Take in that feeling and let it fuel your intention to be alive in your body.

Holding Our Fragile Body with Tenderness

Being alive in a body means opening to uncertainty and vulnerability. We know from our own experience that our body is changing moment by moment and that we have only limited control over how this process unfolds. How do we respond to that truth? Can we still find joy and meaning in our lives when our body hurts, when we get sick, when it ages? Can we continue to love our body when we feel it has let us down? Can we hold it with the tenderness of compassion?

A friend of mine, Karen, called one day to ask if I was free to take a walk in the nearby park. Her little girl was in daycare for a few hours, so this would be a good time. As we walked, our meandering conversation turned to our relationship to our bodies, and she ended up telling me an unexpected story about herself. "As a little girl playing with my dolls, I dreamed of having children when I grew up. And when I was a teenager babysitting my neighbor's baby boy, 'being a mother' felt completely natural to me." But when Karen got married, assuming that having a family would come easily, she was taken by surprise.

"Miscarriages," she said. "I had two of them. And each one was devastating."

Karen told me she had greeted her first pregnancy with utter delight. "I felt elated. I was a mother goddess. Everything felt perfect. I didn't care if I was nauseous, it was an honor to have life growing inside me. Then one night I had a vivid dream. The only thing I remembered when I woke up was the word "ACCEPT," written in really big letters. I wondered what that meant. A few days later when my uterus started contracting, I knew what that dream was about. Losing that baby was harder than anything I'd ever gone through before. Darkness came over me, like being in a hollow cave. My womb was empty. All of my dreams about having a joyous life with this baby were gone. That little being, that spirit, all of it was gone. The grief was unbelievably huge." Her husband was caring and wanted to help, but Karen just wanted to be alone. She didn't think anyone could understand that her whole world has just collapsed.

As Karen and I continued walking in the woods together, she told me that taking long walks outside is how she got through it. "Seeing these trees so powerfully rooted in the ground reminds me of that time. Being around them is what helped me find my way back to myself." As she bent to pick up a pine cone on the pathway, she continued her story. "That first miscarriage was sobering. It showed me how fragile life could be.

"It would be a couple of years before Tom and I decided to try again. I did everything I could to prepare my body—I ate well, took long walks, and got good sleep. More and more I treated my body like a temple. I directed lovingkindness to it every day—and to our delight, one day I had a positive pregnancy test." To celebrate, Karen and Tom went camping with some friends. "After a sing-along around the campfire, we all crawled into our tents. I settled into my sleeping bag and started to dose off when all of a sudden, I felt pain in my womb. Once you've had that pain, you know it. Those are not moon-time cramps, they're labor cramps. I lay there feeling my womb contracting, and I felt like I was back in that dark cave again. But this time I knew I wanted to reach out to Tom and not let my pain push him away. I woke him up and we gently held each other for a long time, together experiencing the pain of losing our dream."

My heart ached as Karen continued her story. "That night the word ACCEPT kept coming up in my mind again, and it stayed with me for many days as I took in the loss of this baby too. My whole being longed for that child, and my moment-to-moment practice was opening to that longing, not denying it but remaining present for my grief." Karen said she found it especially hard seeing other women who were pregnant or listening to friends who'd just had babies. "I would feel angry, and sad, and jealous. I kept asking myself *Why them, why not me? What have I done to deserve this?* I wanted to be gracious and happy for them, but instead I'd feel contracted and confused. *Would I ever have a child?*

Would I have my dream? It was challenging to accept how little control I had over my body."

Our bodies don't always do what we want them to do, and many of us have had to grieve what we have lost or what we wish could have been different. When we meet that sense of loss with a tender heart, not denying our feelings but holding them with compassion, we can allow that grief to move through us.

For months Karen struggled to turn back to her body with love, grieving not only the loss of the pregnancy but also the loss of the connection, joy, and aliveness she had experienced in her body. Now it felt closed and tight, as if she was carrying a heavy weight. Waves of grief would come over her at the most unexpected times, like one afternoon when she was grocery shopping and a little girl in the child's seat of someone's cart smiled at her. Unable to hold back her tears, she ran out of the store sobbing. At Thanksgiving dinner, she struggled to open her heart when everyone was sharing what they were grateful for. And sometimes lying in bed at night, she would feel the pain of what she called her "hollow womb." But she began to see that when she allowed the tears to flow and remained present with her body instead of turning against it or abandoning it, she could feel something releasing and opening in her. A feeling of warmth and tenderness would arise in her heart, and afterward her body would feel lighter. Karen was discovering a source of resilience she had not known before, and it was opening her to new possibilities.

One morning, almost a year after the second miscarriage, Karen woke up feeling like doing something she used to love—going to an early-morning yoga class. She put on leggings and a tank top and drove to the studio. Sitting on her mat waiting for the class to start, she felt a shiver of excitement go through her body. As she rhythmically moved through each asana, she could feel her energy awakening. She was back in her body. After that morning, Karen's body and heart continued to heal. She once again began noticing glimmers of joy in her life. She felt her heart expand when she saw little rainbows shining in the drops of water on the trees and bushes when the sun came out after a rainstorm, or when she looked up and saw a flock of geese flying over her house in a perfect triangle formation. Eventually Karen and Tom decided to start the process of adoption, and a year later they received into their arms a baby girl who they named Iris, the Greek word for rainbow, a symbol of hope, promise, and new beginning.

At the end of our conversation, as Karen was about to get into her car to pick up three-year-old Iris, she said, "I used to remember the dates of each of those miscarriages and mark them by lighting a candle. But I don't anymore. Iris is the gift that life has given me, and her presence fills me with the aliveness I was longing for. And I'm grateful to my body for knowing how to care for her."

When we listen to our body and treat it with respect and kindness, not judging or condemning it for its vulnerabilities, a door can open to a new kind of joy. Our "dream" may look different from what we had imagined, but when that door is open, unexpected gifts may reveal themselves.

This openness to possibility can be especially helpful as we face the fragility of our changing bodies as they age. Johanna is eighty-five years old and lives on her own in her artistically decorated house. One day when we were sitting together drinking tea in her yard, I inquired about how she was feeling. She answered honestly: "I'm feeling my age. My energy is not like it used to be. I have new aches and pains here and there. My eyesight is waning, so I can't drive to the farmers market, and I need people to take me to the theater. But the hardest thing is that I can't walk the dogs around the block. I miss all the people I used to see and talk to when I did that."

Johanna had been a fiercely independent woman who never left any item on her long to-do list undone. She'd thought of herself as a dancer swirling from one thing to the next, full of energy, never needing to stop, never needing to ask for help. So, when undeniable signs of aging started to appear, she felt disheartened, and it took her a couple of years to allow herself to slow down. "What has changed now is my awareness of vulnerability," she said. "I am thinking more about what really matters, and suddenly life itself is the most important thing. I'm aware of my body changing, and the fragility of life is tangible. I can almost touch it. I know I have only one life, and it won't last forever."

Johanna paused and looked around at her garden and her house. "There's always lots to do, but I am spending less time feeling I have to be producing or creating or making new things. Everything has slowed down. I have a new relationship to time, realizing that every moment that has passed is gone. I sat in my chair this morning looking out the window, watching the leaves dancing in the breeze and the sunlight playing through them ... simply *being*. That is enough."

Gratitude for Our Body

Take a few moments to settle into your body. Then you might place your hands on your heart or abdomen and ask: What about my body am I grateful for today? What about my body brings me joy? How do I experience aliveness in my body? You might be grateful for your eyes that see the world or for your ears that can hear the voices of loved ones. You might thank your hands for working, creating, cooking, or touching. You might thank your legs for taking you from place to place, for running, climbing, or biking. You might be grateful for everything in your body that is working well and supporting your life. Let yourself bask in the great fortune of being alive in your body and offer it thanks.

The experience of aging can be filled with fear, anguish, frustration, or it can become a time to settle and relax into our days, discovering new ways to enjoy life and cherish the gift of each moment. Savoring the taste of a peach, the sound of the flute through the next-door neighbor's window, or the sensation of our body climbing a flight of stairs, can fill our heart with gratitude. Meeting moments of vulnerability with tenderness, we remain in touch with the wonder of our transient and changing body, the home of our aliveness.

Turning Back from Brokenness

For some of us, being physically mistreated has left us feeling vulnerable, unsafe, and even disconnected from our bodies. This is what brought Amanda in to see me.

"I can't seem to relax anywhere," she began as she sat down. "When I walk down the street, I keep looking around to see if I'm safe, if there is anyone around who might hurt me." Amanda was only in her twenties, but there were deep lines on her forehead and she carried herself as if worn down by many years. "Nothing feels safe to me. Nowhere feels safe. Even here in your office, I'm keeping an eye on the door, just in case I need to get out."

"Living in our body without a sense of ease and comfort can be very painful, Amanda," I offered in support.

"I don't even know what you mean by 'living in my body,'" she responded. "Sometimes I feel like I am about ten feet away, looking back at myself. When that happens, things around me don't feel quite real. I feel like I'm in a bubble and separate from everything."

"I can only imagine how disorienting and scary it must be to feel so disconnected. How long has this been happening?"

Amanda looked down at the floor and then out the window before bringing her eyes back to me. "As far back as I can remember. It's a long story." She looked at me as if to check if I was up for it. I nodded to reassure her that I was ready to listen.

Amanda was born and raised in a small town in Pennsylvania. Her father, who was well respected in their community, had physically abused her starting from when she was still a toddler. After work he often went out to a bar with some of his friends, and when he got home, he would be drunk and out of control. Of all the children in the family, Amanda was the target of his rage. He would yell at her, hit her, sometimes throw or push her against the couch.

"I don't know why, but for some reason he hated my legs," Amanda continued. "He used to kick them and tell me they were fat and ugly. Sometimes he would pull out his belt and throw me across his knees, and I knew what was coming. After the first blow, my mind would go blank, the pain was so sharp. And then I just didn't feel the rest."

For Amanda, this dissociation, her mind disconnecting from her body, is what had allowed her to survive. According to Peter Levine, dissociation is an altered state of consciousness in which people describe feeling out of their body, sometimes seeing themselves from above or through a fog, or disconnected from what is happening in their environment in the present moment. Dissociation, a physiological and psychological process, removes us from an overwhelming situation and frees us from feeling that which is intolerable. In Levine's words, dissociation "makes the unbearable bearable."

"I'm so sorry that happened to you, Amanda. Was anyone there for you when this was happening?"

My Aunt Mary was the only one I could talk to about it. She tried to intervene, but my mother would say, "He's not that bad—Amanda's just a difficult child," and brush aside her concerns.

"What did you do to get through that time?" I asked.

"As soon as I knew how to ride a bike, I would get out of the house, go down to the creek about ten minutes from our house, and sit by the willow tree. That was my safe place. My father couldn't find me there. And I would take books with me. My favorite stories were *Anne of Green Gables* and *Pippi Longstocking*. Those were girls who had their own minds and their own thoughts. I wanted to be just like them. Then, in high school, I joined the cross–country running team. That also gave me a reason to be gone. I would get up early, put on my headset with music, and run for several miles even before school started. Many days I would stay after school for practice. Running took my mind off what was happening at home, and it gave me a way to stay away from my father. But I always had to come back at some point, and the yelling and hitting would start again."

"And all of that abuse has left you feeling disconnected from your body," I said softly. "Can you let yourself imagine for a moment what your life would be like if you healed this trauma from your childhood?"

After a few moments she said, "I could do simple things, like sitting on a beach and reading a book without constantly looking around to see if I am safe. I could fall asleep more easily at night. Maybe I'd do some kind of physical activity that was fun." This sense of who she might be if she shed the layers of trauma would help guide her healing process.

When Amanda returned the following week, I suggested we start the session with a short mindfulness meditation, gently turning our attention to the body. "I know it can be frightening for you to connect with your body, but maybe we could do this together, and you can stop at any point if you need to."

"I am not sure I can do that," she said. "When suggested that we turn our attention to our bodies, my anxiety shot up. My heart started racing. That's how I felt when I was a child, like something bad was just about to happen and I couldn't get away." Tears started rolling down her cheeks.

"Stay with me if you can, Amanda. Let's breathe into that fear that just got touched and hold it with kindness. You might want to put a hand on your heart, or gently hug yourself. Keep breathing and let this wave of emotion move through you. That's all you need to do."

Many trauma survivors, like Amanda, find that turning their attention to their body is challenging and for some almost impossible. Awareness of the body can awaken pain that had been dormant for years, leading to powerful surges of anxiety or anger, or feelings of disconnection or disorientation. While coming back to the body is necessary in order to heal that pain, the process of doing so can itself be frightening and lead to overwhelm and dissociation. This is why it is important to reawaken the body carefully, with kindness and support. Based on Amanda's response to the mindfulness practice, I knew it would be necessary for her to turn to her body with great patience and in a loving environment that could hold any pain that might arise.

Amanda and I spent several weeks strengthening our trust. When I thought she was ready to try connecting with her body again, I suggested that we try a process Peter Levine had designed to help trauma survivors connect with their body and begin feeling safe in it. "This exercise is about gently directing our attention to the sensations we experience when we lightly touch or tap parts of our body. Would you be open to trying that, Amanda? As Peter Levine points out, when we carefully notice what we are experiencing with that safe and gentle touch, we can begin coming home to the body."

Amanda said she'd be willing to try. When she had settled in, I invited her to begin by slowly tapping or massaging the palm of her left hand. "You may notice the roughness or smoothness of your skin, or the warmth of your hand as you touch your palm. What other sensations do you notice, Amanda?"

"Well, it sort of tickles," she said.

"Now when you stop touching your hand, you may notice that you are still feeling sensations in your palm. Maybe tingling or vibrations."

"Yes, I am feeling tingling ... and warmth."

"As you remain aware of those feelings, say to yourself with kindness, *This is my hand, I feel my hand, my hand is part of me, my hand belongs to me.* You can try that now for a few moments." I waited while she did this.

"When you are ready, do the same with the other hand. Feel the sensations there, and repeat those same phrases."

Amanda took a deep breath and began slowly tapping on the palm of her right hand. Then I guided her in continuing the process, tapping her shoulders, her arms, the back of her neck. "As you connect with each part of your body, notice the subtle vibrations or tingling that remain even after you stop tapping. Then you can move on to your chest, and then your stomach and legs."

Amanda was looking a little more relaxed as she continued tapping, but when she got to her thighs, her lips began to quiver. "I can't feel my legs," she said with an edge in her voice. "And when I try to say *These are my legs,* I can't do it. It feels like there's nothing there that is part of me."

"I am here with you, Amanda. It's okay. Let's slow down and take a few deep breaths. This is part of the process."

"I need a moment," she responded softly as she stood up and walked around the room. After a short while she said, "I'm ready to keep going."

"Okay, now you can gently keep tapping on your legs, and this time pay attention to what you are thinking and feeling." After a few moments, Amanda said, "I feel like I am in that room with my father, and he is kicking me. I want to run away. I want to get out."

She suddenly sat up straight, tense, as if she was ready to spring out of her seat. Recognizing that the trauma from that time was still held in Amanda's body, I encouraged her to stay with that urge to run and we would work with it. As Peter Levine points out, imagining ourselves successfully escaping to safety or fighting back in ways we could not do at the time of the experience helps release some of the energy of the trauma that has remained in our body. As we do that, we begin to reclaim our sense of power and agency. That's what I wanted to guide Amanda toward.

"Where do you want to run to, Amanda? Is there some place where you would feel safe again?" I asked.

"I would need to run halfway across the world to feel safe," she answered. "I would need to be that far from my father." She paused and closed her eyes, then said, "Actually, I would run back to my willow tree by the creek."

"You can imagine yourself now running to that special place. Let yourself feel the wind on your face and the temperature of the air." I continued to slowly guide her. "Feel your feet touching the earth as each step meets the ground. Maybe you can hear the sound of the creek flowing past. You can let yourself see your willow tree just up ahead of you. When you come close to it and duck under its long branches, feel the safety of that place. Notice the feeling of the bark as you touch the tree, and let yourself stay there, safe with your tree."

I waited as Amanda's breath grew deep and slow. Her face began to look relaxed in a way I had not seen before. After another long breath, she looked at me, and with a small smile said, "It felt good to run. It has been a long time since I let myself do that, and I was glad to be under my willow tree again."

"And now that you're not trapped in that room with your father and you are able to run, do your legs feel any different?" I asked.

Amanda stroked her thighs. "They're starting to tingle."

"Well, then that was a successful sprint," I said, and we both laughed.

The next time we met, we took a detour away from the pain of the trauma, and Amanda told me stories about her love of running, about the strength she used to feel in her body, the kinship she felt with the girls on her team. At the end of that session, I asked, "Amanda, what would it feel like to take up running again? Instead of running away from your father, you could run with the intention of befriending your legs, of taking them back as part of your body."

Amanda smiled. "Interesting to think about that."

"Yes, this could be a big step for you. If you do decide to go out running, keep paying attention to your body. Feel your feet touching the ground. Feel the air on your skin as you move. Notice your breath as it changes."

As Amanda was leaving, I was happy to hear her say that maybe she was ready to get her body back.

Amanda did start running again, every morning making her way up the hill near her house. At our next session she told me how much she enjoyed being out there early in the morning. "I love seeing the sunrise and hearing the birds. As I run, I've been repeating those phrases to myself: *These are my legs. I can feel my legs. My legs belong to me.* I can't feel them all the time, but I really like saying those words. They're hopeful."

Then one day Amanda arrived for her session excited to tell me what had happened. "One morning last week when I was out running, I began to feel the rhythm in the movement of my legs, and it was like they were connected to me again. The next thing I knew, I was sobbing. The feelings were so strong that I had to stop running. I dropped down on my knees and cried and cried—for that little girl in me who was so scared, for the humiliation I felt when my father kicked my legs and told me they were chubby and short, for the woman in me who felt disconnected from her own body for so many years. I stayed there for a while, sitting on the hillside as the sun slowly rose. And when I started running home, I felt them—I felt the power in my legs, inside them, right through them."

Healing trauma is a gradual process that unfolds as we gently return to our body with care, touching on the pain, the numbness, or the discomfort, and releasing it. As we turn back from the brokenness and slowly heal the pain of the past, the symptoms of trauma begin to subside. We once again live in our body without fear, and we trust it as we venture into the world, knowing we can make wise choices that keep us safe.

If you are in an abusive situation and are not safe, please reach out for help to a friend, a family member, or an agency that can support you.
National Domestic Violence Hotline 1-800-799-7233. Service in multiple languages.
National Sexual Assault Hotline 1-800-656-4673. Or online at rainn.org.

Reclaiming Our Sexuality

Sexual energy is part of our aliveness, part of living in a body, part of the sacred nature of our being. Whether we identify as cisgender or transgender, whether we are heterosexual, bisexual, pansexual, or asexual, all of us have a relationship to our sexuality, and it is one of the main ways we define ourselves. Our social, economic, political, religious, and cultural contexts might affect our choices, behaviors, and attitudes about our sexuality, but no matter what these might be, part of our journey back to ourselves is about accepting and celebrating our sexuality with openness, curiosity, and love. We may choose to express our sexuality through lovemaking and self-pleasuring, through pregnancy and giving birth, through creative expression, or may transmute it in spiritual practices, but whatever our personal relationship is to this natural energy, sexuality is part of us, and without it, we would not have been born.

Some of us discovered sexual energy at a young age when we first felt those delightful sensations. Many of us experienced a surge of sexual energy in our adolescence when our sexual attractions and desires got projected onto our friends, random people we saw on the street, or onto movie stars. Some of us may not have felt the first awakening of sexual desire until adulthood, when we met someone with whom we could share that energy. Some may not discover the depth of their passion until they are elders. And many of us, at points in our lives or in certain contexts, might deliberately choose to abstain from sexual activity. Nuns and monks in the Buddhist and Christian traditions may choose to dedicate their life energy to their spiritual practices, feeling fully alive and content without being sexually active. While engaging our sexual energy is a powerful sacred path to aliveness, it is a choice and not a necessity for being whole and complete.

For most of us, our interest in sexuality and the level of our sexual desire fluctuates and changes from day to day and throughout our life.

We might feel a surge of libido when we ovulate. We may feel sexually excited after we go dancing, or after we watch a sex scene in a movie or read one in a book. We might feel a drop in sexual desire when we are tired or upset, or when we don't feel loved or emotionally safe. Some of us notice sexual desire diminishing when we are in a safe long-term love relationship, and some feel the opposite, finally free to be fully sexual. And at times, any of us might feel we would rather read a book or get a good night's sleep.

Our sexuality can be a source of joy, bliss, creativity, and connection, but it can also be a source of pain, confusion, guilt, or shame. If we have been shamed for our sexual desire, our sexual fantasies, or our sexual behaviors, we might believe that something is wrong with the way we feel or act in this area of our lives. We might hold ourselves back from expressing ourselves sexually, hide our body, limit our vision of what is possible for us, and try to fit into the mold of what we were told is right or moral, abandoning ourselves by abandoning our sexuality. We might also abandon ourselves by having sex out of obligation when we would rather not, or when we go silent instead of saying *no* to sexual advances that are nonconsensual. We abandon ourselves if we don't speak up when we have been assaulted, fearing we will rock the boat, lose our jobs, or fearing we will be blamed for being the one who is at fault.

We abandon ourselves when our self-worth gets attached to our ability to reach sexual climax, to being a virgin, or to the number of sexual partners we have had. And we abandon ourselves when we use our sexual energy in ways that are not careful or sensitive and end up hurting ourselves or others. Recognizing we have abandoned ourselves in any of these ways awakens us, and we begin to turn back by healing ourselves and reclaiming our wholeness.

Gail came to see me because, as she put it, "something feels off in my sexual energy." She told me she was married, the mother of a two-year-old girl, and that she had a job as the lead scientist at a research lab. Her life was full to the brim. "Before Sheila was born, Sean and I had a thriving sexual relationship. But after she arrived, my libido fell flat.

At first, we were both so enamored with the baby that we got a lot of those happy connecting-hormones just from being with her. I thought it was 'normal' to bond with your baby and be less interested in sex, at least for some time. But now it's almost two years since she was born and my sex drive is still gone, it's just not there. Sean says things like, 'You like the baby more than you care about me.' He pretends like he's joking, but he's pretty frustrated and has started pulling away emotionally. I'm afraid I'm going to lose him."

For a variety of reasons, women can find themselves going through a change in the level of their sexual energy. This can come from overworking, from changing hormones, from stress, or could be the side effect of medications or a result of illness. Change in our level of sexual desire is in itself not a problem. But when we judge ourselves for it, we find ourselves in the downward spiral of self-abandonment.

Gail's voice was trembling as she asked, "Is there something wrong with me? Will I ever get my passion back?"

"This is all quite normal," I assured her. "Many women lose their sexual desire for some time after they give birth. And we all go through cycles of wanting and not wanting to be intimate with someone. What you feel in your body today is your own truth." I saw a small tear well up in the corner of her eye.

"If you were to turn to your body right now, what would it be telling you? What is it asking for? What does it need in order to feel alive?"

She smiled. "It's simple. What I need is not sex. I need a good night's sleep. Maybe a few in a row. Between work and family, I need some alone time. As much as I love Sheila and Sean, I am "all touched out." We brainstormed a few options, and Gail decided to talk with Sean to see if he would be willing to be the one to put Sheila to bed for a few nights. "And this one might be a little harder for him—I want to sleep in the guest room those nights."

When Gail returned for her next session, she did look more rested. "I did it!" she said with delight. "I arranged those three nights alone in that other room. The first night, I laid down on the bed and spread my body out as if to say *This is my space, this is my body!* For the first two nights, I was so tired, I just fell asleep within minutes. But by the third night, I started imagining Sean and Sheila in the other bedroom together, and my heart yearned to be back with them. Very quietly I tiptoed in and snuggled into bed. Sean put his arms around me, and we fell asleep." Gail let out a long sigh of relief. "We still haven't started having sex again, but that little break I took seemed good for both of us."

Gail spent the next month caring for her body. She made sure to leave work on time, she asked her mother for help with Sheila, and she went back to making herself green smoothies in the morning. She started being more available to snuggle with Sean and watch a TV show at night after Sheila went to sleep.

"Now that you are so beautifully caring for your body, and you feel more connected to Sean, let's see if there is a way you can enjoy connecting with him sexually again. Can you recall a time with Sean when your erotic energy was alive and flowing with ease?"

Gail thought for minute, and then a big smile spread across her face. "It was early in our relationship. Sean and I had gone to see our favorite band playing in a nearby town. This was not long after we got married. We danced all night and then camped out in the middle of a big field. The stars were bright and there were fireflies everywhere. Making love was magical and like we had entered a sacred space. I felt so open and passionate and fully alive. I still cherish that night."

"What a beautiful memory. Maybe that can be a clue about a way you two can reconnect again."

Gail sighed with relief when she sat down at the beginning of her next session. "I think we're back," she said with a smile. "I asked my mother to watch Sheila, and Sean and I took ourselves out for a hike and then camped out at what used to be one of our favorite places to go together. That night we found our way back to each other's bodies ... and hearts. We've made an arrangement with Grandma and Sheila so that we can take this kind of time for ourselves more often. And it looks like everybody is happy with this arrangement."

Reclaiming our sexuality is a practice of listening to our body and learning what it is asking for. It is about learning what awakens our sexual desire, what shuts it down, and choosing when and if we wish to be sexually active. With that knowledge, we turn back to ourselves and reclaim our vitality.

For Gail, life circumstances had gotten in the way of a healthy and easeful expression of her sexuality. But for Anne, another client of mine, the challenge was much deeper. She had grown up in a very religious family that devoutly followed the rules and practices of their faith. Although they never spoke to Anne about sex, she discovered her own sexual energy early in life and secretly enjoyed that pleasure long before she knew what the word "masturbation" meant. But when she was ten years old, in her youth group at church, she started hearing a different attitude toward sex, and slogans like "Save yourself for marriage" and "True love waits," were making it clear that sexual pleasure was a sin and should be repressed. She shut down any sense of herself as a woman with sexual feelings.

But when Anne was in her last year of college, something happened that turned her world around. She fell in love with a woman in one of her classes, and all that powerful sexual energy awakened in her again. This opened a deep rift inside her. While one part of her loved the possibility of sharing sexual pleasure with Beth, the teachings of the religion she grew up with were still deeply ingrained in her. Not only would loving Beth mean having sex outside of marriage, but it would be sex with a woman.

Anne came to see me to try and make sense of all the thoughts and feelings that were swirling around in her mind and heart. "When Beth and I met at school, we liked each other a lot," she began. "We started spending time together, studying in her apartment off campus. Then one night, sitting in the armchair in her living room, I watched her walk across the room, and I felt a surge of energy rising right through the center of my body. My heart just flew open. I loved Beth ... and I also loved her body. I loved her curves, I loved her lips and her hips, I loved her breasts and her buttocks. We ended up kissing passionately, and I felt transported to another world. That night back at home, the guilt started pouring in. I'm feeling completely lost. I have fallen in love with a woman and my body is on fire, and all of this is going against everything I learned at church and at home. I don't know if this is the happiest time of my life, or if I am about to lose everything I ever had."

"I can hear that this relationship has opened such a profound sense of aliveness in you, Anne. Let's explore some of that conflict you're feeling inside and see where it might lead to in your heart."

Anne took a few deep breaths. "Yes, that is why I'm here."

Anne and I spent some time looking at the messages she had received from her family and church, what those beliefs had meant to her, and what they meant now. As she worked through the fear and the guilt about sex that she had carried since her youth group, she began to reclaim the ease and joy she had known in her body as a young girl. As we worked together, she and Beth did begin developing a beautiful sexual relationship, and then one day she told me she had realized something that was transforming her relationship to her own body. "I was noticing how much I appreciated Beth's body, and suddenly I thought, *If I can love that body that much, I can surely love my own.* It was life-changing!"

As Anne reclaimed her love for her body, she also fully claimed the freedom to express her sexuality in the way that felt alive and right for her. In our final session, she said, "Turning back to my body has not only been about opening to the beauty and ecstasy of sexuality. For me the real triumph has been seeing that letting go of all that fear and confusion has allowed me to reclaim the deepest and most raw core elements of my being."

Reclaiming our sexuality means not only knowing our body and how it wants to express itself but also knowing how to create safe relationships and environments in which our erotic nature can be discovered and expressed. In our culture we are waking up to the importance of communicating our needs, our desires, and our preferences. We are learning how to have conversations about intimacy and sex. We are learning that consent is not a choice but a necessary ingredient for sexual relationships. We are finding an authentic voice inside us that expresses the truth about our bodies and how to hold them with care and love. We are finding the courage to speak up for the safety and dignity of ourselves and all women. Drawing on the wisdom of the body, we can create an agreement with ourselves to stay mindful, loving, and kind as we allow sexual energy to move through us.

Opening to our sexuality is one way to reclaim the power and joy of our bodies and awaken beauty, confidence, openness, and ease. When a woman's body is well-loved, I see a smile that I like to call "the after-lovemaking smile," a sweet sense of presence and fulfillment in her body. As we enter the sanctuary of our body and take back our sexuality as a sacred part of us, we reclaim our aliveness and our sense of connection to life.

Turning Back to Loving Our Body

Loving our body is a homecoming, and as Anne found, sometimes someone else can help awaken us to its beauty. This is especially important when we have dismissed or disregarded our body or forgotten how to love it. Several months after Janet and I had stopped working together, she called to make an appointment. When she stepped into my office, I could see that something about her was different. She seemed to be more present, and she actually looked taller. She told me she had continued the mindful eating practice and had begun over time to feel better about her body. And then something unexpected happened—she met Eli.

They were both at a peace rally and had laughed and talked with each other for hours. They exchanged numbers, and over the next few months, their ease and connection grew. When they spent their first night together, Janet told me she'd felt safe with Eli but "I felt so vulnerable and sensitive about being a big woman that I insisted on keeping my T-shirt on to cover my belly. Eli was very sweet and understanding about it. I think he might have known what was going on for me. Then the next time he stayed over and I kept that shirt on, he asked very gently if he might touch my belly. I pulled back. 'No!' I said to him sharply and told him he could touch me anywhere else but not there." Janet said she had surprised herself for having such a strong response, but Eli had listened and gently stroked her hair and her back until she fell asleep. "He was being kind, but I just felt so self-conscious and vulnerable … and scared."

Guarding her body like this went on for a few more weeks. And then one night Eli told her how much he loved her and that he loved her body, her whole body, and wished that she could open to that love for herself. He asked her if she would be willing to sit in front of a mirror with him and see herself as he saw her. Her heart pounding, Janet looked in his eyes and could see that he meant what he was saying. Moved by his love, she nodded. Eli put his hand on her cheek for a moment, then asked if she would wait in the kitchen while he prepared the room for her. When he led her back in, Janet's eyes filled with tears. The full-length mirror was surrounded by candles and flowers, and there were soft pillows for them to sit on. Eli had created a sacred space for her.

Still in her shirt, Janet sat down next to him, and Eli gently asked if she would look in the mirror and name the parts of her body that she could love. Feeling a little embarrassed, Janet started by naming her brown eyes, and then her full lips. She told him the story about baking bread and how that had allowed her to love her hands. "But I still don't …" she began, and Eli gently brought her back to his question. "You can take your time, Janet, there is no rush. What other parts of your body can you love?" She paused and felt a wave of fear pass through her. "It wasn't easy," she told me, "but I took off my big T-shirt, put my hand on my belly and whispered, 'This too I can love.'" The pain of hating her belly for so many years flowed out with her tears. Janet reached for Eli's hand and placed it over hers, loving and claiming this part of her body again.

"That evening with Eli changed me," she said. "That was the first time I had ever experienced loving all of myself. I was sitting there with him, seeing my body in the mirror surrounded by candlelight, and no matter what size or shape it was—it is—I can hold it with love."

We may not have an "Eli" to bring us back to the beauty of our body just as it is, but we can open our heart to our own uniqueness with gratitude and love. We might even sit in front of our own mirror, name the parts of our body we love, and then slowly open to the parts that we have left behind. We can listen to what our body needs and respond with kindness and care. We can appreciate and celebrate the joy and aliveness our body offers us. We can each find our own unique way to turn back to our body, get to know it, befriend it, and create an intimate relationship with it. We might turn back through mindfulness practice, paying attention moment by moment to sensations in the body, noticing subtle vibrations, the sensations of movement, and the experience of stillness. We might turn back by seeing and feeling the beauty, strength, and resilience of our body. And we can turn back by celebrating our body, caring for it, and using it in ways that enliven it—walking, hiking, swimming, biking.

As Amanda continued her morning run in the hills near her house, she discovered again how much she enjoyed being physically active. As she learned to live again in her body, her sense of safety grew stronger. So, when a friend invited her to join the women's team for the annual "dragon–boat race" on a local lake, Amanda did not hesitate. Being with a group of women taking on a rigorous challenge appealed to her. With each practice her muscles grew stronger, as did the friendships she was developing with the others on the team. Learning to join with them, rowing together as one, opened her to love and trust the safety of her own body.

Anne and Beth invited friends to their beautiful marriage celebration on a mountaintop. Not long after, they began arrangements with a sperm bank for Anne to get pregnant. They both loved hearing the baby's heartbeat and stroking Anne's firm belly. Beth was at Anne's side through the pain and euphoria of labor as Anne surrendered to the powerful waves of energy moving through her. And when she felt the burning sensation of her baby's head crowning, she also felt Beth's hands reaching to catch their baby, and together they welcomed little Lia into the world. For Anne this celebration was also about her courage to love who she loved, no longer held back by beliefs or doctrines but fully claiming her own sexuality and the freedom to express it.

Turning back to loving our body is an essential part of our journey back to ourselves. We welcome our body into our hearts by experiencing its vitality through our senses, by listening to what it longs for, and by trusting its wisdom in response. We honor and respect its needs for nourishment, exercise, touch, and rest. Taking care of our body in these ways brings us home to ourselves. Stretching our arms and legs in bed when we wake up in the morning, coming back from a run with our heart still pounding, making love, enjoying flavorful food—these are all moments of being in our body with aliveness, joy, and gratitude. When we dwell in our bodies with love and appreciation, our hearts open and we turn back to ourselves, to all of who we are.

CHAPTER SIX

Living with Spaciousness: Turning Back to Center

Our emotions are a rich and colorful expression of our hearts, part of the tapestry of our lives. They can be intense, like fierce anger in response to injustice, or exuberance when we ride our bicycle down a hill and feel the wind on our face. Or they can be subtle, like the warmth that arises in us when we see a newborn baby, or the wave of longing or delight we feel when we hear a song we love. Some emotions feel like little ripples on the water and some like a tidal wave. Some are pleasant and some are painful, but they are all part of our human experience. While our emotions can guide us, protect us from harm, and enrich our lives, they can also at times become overwhelming, causing us to hurt ourselves or hurt others, leading us into the downward spiral of self–abandonment.

Taking a moment to notice our emotions, we can see that they are arising as sensations in the body interconnected with a stream of thoughts arising in the mind. For instance, when we feel love for someone we care about, it might arise as warmth in our heart and a sensation of expansion in our chest, along with remembering what we most appreciate about that person. We may engage in activities we enjoy, or when we feel happy at seeing the happiness of others, we may experience pleasant sensations in our body. We may feel a tenderness in our heart when we see others in pain and the wish arises to alleviate their suffering. We may feel the tightness of anxiety in our abdomen when something in our environment feels dangerous, and we begin thinking about how we can find safety. We might feel heat rising with anger when we have been hurt, violated, or disrespected, and we begin imagining how we might fight back. We may feel the ache of grief as we think of a loved one we have lost, and we remember the beautiful times we spent together.

Being mindful and aware of the thoughts and sensations that make up our emotions allows us to stay open to whatever we are feeling and remain centered. This is especially important when strong difficult emotions arise. Even in the face of sorrow or anger, we can remain grounded and skillful in our responses. Anchored in awareness of our body and mind, we can allow waves of emotion to rise within us, naturally reach their peak, and then subside. Living with this balanced state of mind is what psychiatrist Daniel Siegel, the author of *Mindsight* and *The Developing Mind,* calls being in the "Window of Tolerance." In this state we remain mindful of whatever is arising in our field of awareness. Open, spacious, and present, we are able to "tolerate" whatever emotional state arises, staying curious and balanced, in touch with our wise and compassionate self.

When we are in our Window of Tolerance, day-to-day chores and stresses are manageable. We approach problems with clear thinking, creativity, and flexibility. When circumstances arise that bring up strong reactions, we make wise and balanced choices in how we respond. If a fly lands on our cheek and we feel a wave of annoyance, we just brush it off without getting angry or upset. If we find our housemate's backpack left in the middle of the living room (again), we notice the thoughts of judgment and blame arising in our mind, take a breath, pick up the backpack and set it aside, knowing we can talk with them about it later, if necessary.

When we are well rested, well fed, and have had physical exercise, our Window of Tolerance tends to be wider and we have more capacity to be present for life. When we have had the right amount of social engagement and support, and also have had time to be with ourselves and to unwind, we are more able to flow with life and adjust to changing needs and circumstances. When we have a regular spiritual practice, such as meditation or prayer, or we engage in centering disciplines, such as yoga or martial arts, we are more able to meet life with spaciousness and compassion. When our Window of Tolerance is wide, we can respond to challenging situations thoughtfully and with equanimity.

However, as we all know, we're not always in that balanced emotional state. There are times when we are overcome by difficult emotions and can get lost in them. According to Daniel Siegel, our ability to stay within our Window of Tolerance varies depending upon circumstances in our life. When our body is stressed because we are exhausted, hungry, physically unwell, or facing a hormonal wave, we may be more reactive. Or we may reach our limit and lash out when we are overworked or feel alone and unsupported. We might be consumed by anxiety or depression when we don't have enough money for food or medications, when we live in inadequate housing, or when we are unemployed. We may find ourselves thrown out of balance when our inner reserves have been used up and we feel depleted, or when we are angry or scared, hurt or humiliated. Especially if we live with unhealed trauma, our Window of Tolerance tends to be narrow and our ability to cope with stress is limited.

In any of these situations, we leave the Window of Tolerance and lose our sense of balance and equanimity. We have less capacity to be mindful, open, and spacious with the emotions that are arising in response to what we are experiencing. We struggle to think clearly, feel less able to care for ourselves or others, and it doesn't take much to push us over the edge. That fly lands on our cheek, and we explode in anger. Or that backpack is left in the middle of the living room floor and we "lose" it, spewing out blame and resentment. Or in contrast to those hyperarousal reactions, we might fall into a downward spiral. Our supervisor offers feedback on our work, and we withdraw and shut down, feeling ashamed and hopeless.

Outside the Window of Tolerance, we find ourselves in one of two states—hyperarousal or hypoarousal (see diagram.) When we are swept away by anger or overcome with panic or anxiety and we want to fight or run away, we are in hyperarousal. Like a deer in headlights, we may freeze for a moment and then launch into reaction, fighting or fleeing. In these states our body and mind react instantly to whatever might be a real or perceived threat. Our heart rate increases, our breath gets faster, and we might start sweating.

In response to overwhelming situations that often have developed over time, we might instead find ourselves feeling shut down, fatigued, depressed, or experiencing dissociation. This is hypoarousal. Our heart rate might slow down, we may have difficulty concentrating, and we collapse into numbness or indifference, withdrawing from activities we usually enjoy, and avoiding people we love.

Overcome by anxiety and anger in hyperarousal or feeling pulled down by exhaustion or depression in hypoarousal, we speak and act in ways that are not aligned with who we know ourselves to be. Lost in difficult emotions, we forget our love for ourselves and our connection to others. Tossed around by waves of emotion, we lose sight of our capacity for mindfulness, compassion, and equanimity—the rafts that can bring us back to shore.

Hyperarousal: High Emotional Energy

Angry – Anxious – Stressed – Reactive
Hypervigilant – Overwhelmed – Irritable
Aggressive – Frustrated
Worrying – Panicked – Easily Startled

Window of Tolerance

Open – Spacious – Present for Life
Calm – Connected – Able to Self–Soothe
Alert – Engaged – Loving – Compassionate

Hypoarousal: Low Emotional Energy

Fatigued – Difficulty Focusing or Concentrating
Withdrawn – Reclusive – Lacking Interest
Depressed –Ashamed – Hopeless
Dissociated – Shut Down – Numb

Figure 1. The Window of Tolerance Model by Dr. Daniel Siegel

When we find ourselves outside the Window of Tolerance, we can learn to reach out to others for support and find ways to care for ourselves that help us find safe ground again. With mindfulness we can be aware of painful emotions and allow them to move through us without judgment or reaction. Sending ourselves metta can remind us to hold ourselves with kindness and understanding. And touching our pain with compassion, we can turn back to center and engage with all that life is offering us.

> ### Exploring Your Window of Tolerance
>
> ~
>
> Let yourself remember a time when you felt anger, rage, or high waves of anxiety, the state of hyperarousal. Or a time when you were in a state of hypoarousal, feeling depressed, lethargic, or disconnected from life. What were you feeling in your body at that time? What thoughts were going through your mind? What helped you return to your Window of Tolerance? Maybe you talked with a friend, went for a walk, or wrote in your journal. Maybe you sat down and meditated, or you did yoga or Qigong. What did you feel in your body, your mind, and your heart when you returned to the Window of Tolerance? Take a moment to appreciate the inner wisdom that can always guide you back to balance and spaciousness.

Lost in Reactivity

Colleen found that the lovingkindness and self–compassion practices she learned in the women's circle were helping her be less hard on herself when she lost her temper or was impatient. But as her pregnancy progressed, she once again found herself snapping at Jacob, even over little things. And not only at him. One night the college students next door were partying late, and she stormed over to their house and told them to turn down the music or she would call the police. And she was often impatient with customer service people on the telephone. "I feel so bad afterward," she said when she called me to ask if she could schedule a therapy session with me. "I'm beginning to worry I'll take my anger out on my child, just like my mother did when I was growing up." She said she desperately needed to learn how to calm her reactive mind. I hoped that we could build on the mindfulness practices Colleen had already learned so that she could begin catching her emotional reactions before they took over. We made an appointment for the following week.

"You can't believe what is happening," she said, as soon as she walked into the room. "I'm doing it again. I try, I really try," she went on, the words tumbling out of her mouth. "I try to not raise my voice, but my anger comes spilling out. I feel like there's a "monster woman" in me and I don't know what to do to stop her." Colleen dropped onto the couch. "Same old, same old," she said. "The other night I blamed Jacob for something, I don't even remember what, and started yelling at him. He got hurt, I apologized, but I know it will happen again. Something needs to change. I am ruining my life, and I'm going to ruin my family too."

Her face was flushed, her breathing fast and shallow. Colleen was clearly outside her Window of Tolerance. Knowing that moving our bodies can help release some of that excess energy and regulate emotion, I suggested we go for a walk. Outside we were met by the fresh winter air. We walked around the block a couple of times, not talking much. After about twenty minutes, Colleen's steps slowed down. She looked at me with a smile. "I think I can go back inside now. Maybe a cup of tea?"

Settled back in my office, each of us holding a warm mug in our hands, I handed her a copy of Daniel Siegel's diagram. "That middle section, the Window of Tolerance, identifies the emotions we feel when we are fully alive, present, and balanced in the face of whatever is arising in our life."

"I do know that feeling," Colleen said. "That's when I find myself singing. Jacob and I are getting along. I remember what I love about him. I'm just doing the day. Life feels uneventful in a good way. If anything comes up, I can handle it without turning it into a crisis."

"I love that you already know how it feels to be centered. But when you fall out of the Window of Tolerance, it sounds to me like you go into hyperarousal," I said, pointing out that area of the diagram.

"Yes, I'm sure familiar with these states," she said, looking at the list.

"In this emotional state, our heart starts pounding and we might feel like we can't sit still. Sometimes we feel waves of anxiety that seem as high as mountains. We might notice a strong surge of anger rising in us, and we can feel like we're losing control. That is when even the best-intentioned mothers raise their voices, spank their children, slam doors, or throw things across the room."

Colleen sighed. "That was my mother."

"Yes, you talked about her in the women's circle," I said. "From your story I gather that she, too, left her Window of Tolerance quite often and went into fight response. It happens to many of us when we are stretched beyond our limit." Colleen nodded. "And as you know," I continued, "hyperarousal is an all-encompassing experience. Sometimes we don't even know what started it. But whether we're feeling it ourselves or experiencing it from someone else, our body, mind, and heart are suddenly on high alert."

"That's what happens when I get angry at Jacob," Colleen said. "My heart starts racing and I can't take a full breath. I start saying all those hurtful things." She paused for a moment. "I get it. When I'm outside my Window of Tolerance, the monster woman comes out. She can be very scary and can hurt other people. I get scared by her myself."

We continued exploring what happened to Colleen when she was in hyperarousal, and I reassured her that she could learn how to regulate those strong emotions even when she was feeling highly reactive. "During this next week, you can take a first step in the process. Start noticing when the monster woman comes up, what allows that to happen, and what you're feeling in your body at those times."

As Colleen was leaving, she said, "Can I please take this drawing of the Window of Tolerance with me? I want to show it to Jacob and put it on the refrigerator." I was glad it could serve as a useful reminder, knowing that she would probably be facing the monster woman again.

Pausing at the "About–to–Moment"

"Well, that was interesting," Colleen said when she walked into my office the following week. "I got to know the monster woman a lot better." I was glad to see that she seemed a little more grounded and relaxed. She eased down onto the couch, adjusted her top over her growing pregnant belly, and went on. "I noticed that most of the time she came up in me when I was short of sleep or when I hadn't eaten. Some little thing would happen, the anger would start rising, and I would lose it. If Jacob wasn't there, I'd start yelling at the cat if she got under my feet, or I'd even yell at myself. But a couple of times this week I actually noticed the sensations coming up in my body, like you suggested. So instead of getting all caught in the feelings, I found that if I could just stay aware of them, often the wave of anger would pass. But sometimes the emotion was still too strong, it would get the best of me, and the monster woman would win."

"Noticing those sensations even once in a while and being able to stop yourself from acting on them is progress, Colleen. As you have seen, there is a moment between the impulse to yell and when you start yelling. I've heard Joseph Goldstein call this the "about–to–moment." That is when the phone rings and we are about to reach for it, or the moment when we are about to take a bite of food, or when we are about to speak. In the about–to–moment, we can pause and become aware of what we are about to do or say. But when we are overcome by difficult emotions, we often don't even notice the intention to say harsh words, to raise our voice, or to shame or blame others. We just say or do what comes to mind without pausing or stopping to consider the impact of our actions.

"That's exactly what happens to me." Colleen jumped in. "The impulse to start yelling comes up in me, and before I know it, the words just come out. I'm definitely outside of the Window of Tolerance."

"When emotions are high, we act out of the momentum of habit. But pausing at the about-to-moment and noticing the emotions and the intention that is arising with them, we can choose how to act. When you are about to start yelling, in that pause you can ask yourself 'What is happening in my mind? What am I feeling in my body? What is my intention? Do I really want to hurt Jacob … or the cat?' Pausing at the about-to-moment is like standing at a crossroads and choosing between two paths. One is the path of reactivity, the path of self-abandonment. The other is the path of love and compassion. When we pause, we claim the possibility of refraining from harm, and we get to choose the path that will lead us back to ourselves."

I could see that Colleen was listening carefully. "Does that mean I don't have to lash out every time a surge of anger rises in me? I don't have to stomp off or blame Jacob. I can pause and not react. Easier said than done."

"Yes, pausing at the about-to-moment is not always easy to do. When we are outside our Window of Tolerance, it takes a strong resolve—and practice—to stop the momentum of the reaction that is arising in us. In the pause, we can notice our thoughts and feelings, and with mindfulness and compassion we can remain present with those feelings, not denying them and not acting them out. We can wait until the reaction subsides before we act or speak."

"Sometimes I have tried to take a few breaths, and nothing changes. The situation stays the same, and I'm still raging," Colleen said with desperation in her voice.

"For most of us it takes more than just a few breaths to come back to ourselves. We need to allow the stress hormones to drain out of the body. Research shows that it takes about twenty to thirty minutes for adrenaline levels to decline. During that time, you could take a walk, water the plants, make yourself a cup of tea, and mostly hold yourself in kindness. When you feel the tension leave your body and your mind starts to relax, you are ready to make wiser choices and act skillfully with compassion."

As we practice pausing at the about–to–moment, we get better at recognizing when we have left the Window of Tolerance, and we can turn back to center. We can pause in the middle of an argument, or just after it begins. And over time we can pause at the about–to–moment before we even leave the Window of Tolerance, before we utter harsh words, before we become defensive, before we cause harm. No matter at what point we wake up, we reap the benefits of stopping the forward momentum of reactivity.

A couple of months after Colleen and I had started working on managing her reactivity, in a meeting of the women's circle, she proudly told us that she had begun recognizing the warning signs signaling that she was about to cross the threshold out of her Window of Tolerance. She said she could feel the first inkling of her heart rate getting faster, her breathing pattern changing, and the first blaming thoughts rising in her mind. Being aware of those changes in her body and her mind, combined with an intention to not cause harm, she had begun to change her pattern of lashing out with anger when she felt stressed.

Even though the power of habit can be strong, with practice we can interrupt the reactivity that arises when we are overwhelmed, and we can turn back to our center. Pausing protects us from abandoning ourselves, giving us the time to regain our ability to think clearly and to choose wholesome actions. This is the gift we give ourselves and others—the practice of remaining centered even in the midst of upheavals in our lives.

> ### The Pause
>
> ~
>
> Choose an activity that you typically perform every day, something simple like putting on your shoes. Set the intention to pause at the about-to-moment. When you are about to reach for your shoes, bring your attention to your body and mind and notice the urge to act. As you are about to step into each shoe, pause and notice your intention and your feelings. After you have practiced this for a while, try bringing the pause to an emotionally charged situation. When anger or fear arise, notice what is happening in your body and mind. Maybe you are about to speak harshly, or maybe you are preparing to slam the door and stomp out of the house. Take a breath and notice that you have a choice in that moment. How does this awareness change your behavior?

Pulled Down by Exhaustion and Depression

I was in line for our weekly potluck at Cayuga Lake when a young woman behind me introduced herself. "Hi, I'm Melanie. This is a lovely event. Have you been here before? This is the first time for me." Within a few minutes we were deep into conversation, learning about each other's lives. She told me she had just moved back to the East Coast from California, where she had been working for the past few years as a computer programmer at a company in Silicon Valley. She was here in Ithaca now because she'd wanted to be closer to her family who were living on a farm a couple of hours north. "Growing up on that farm was magical and the best childhood I could have ever asked for," she told me as we were filling our plates from the bountiful spread.

Melanie still seemed to carry some of that magic she was referring to in her childhood, and I wanted to know more. We found a place to sit, and she continued. "We had a lot of freedom to come and go, so we were often out playing in the woods, swimming in the lake, sledding in the wintertime. My grandma lived nearby and so did lots of cousins, uncles, and aunts. Of course, my brother and sister and I all had chores to do, collecting eggs, helping my dad with milking, helping my mom with the garden and stuff around the house. She was always busy, cooking for everyone—the family, the hired hands, the neighbors, and for my grandma. So, there was lots to do every day, but on Sunday morning we all took off work and went to church together. Mom would put on her best dress and a hat and lipstick. She looked beautiful. She was a happy woman."

"You seem happy like her. Do you take after your mother?" I asked.

"Kind of," she said, "but I was different from her. As a child, I loved to make up stories in my head. Sometimes I would get lost in one of them in the middle of my chores and just get up and go write in my notebook. My mother never failed to find me. I couldn't tell if she was truly angry or just pretending to be, but the message was clear—work comes first! Later, when I was supposed to be sleeping, sometimes I'd go back to writing my story, using a flashlight under the covers." Melanie laughed, remembering.

"But I gave all that up when I went to college. Getting a degree in IT made more sense, and it definitely has paid off. I had a good job in California, and I must have got great references from them because a start-up tech company here snatched me right up. But I haven't had much time to meet people yet. This new job takes a lot of work."

"I lead a women's circle that meets once a month. Maybe you would like to check it out as a way to connect with some wise and wonderful women who live in the area?" She was immediately interested. "I'll somehow find the time to do it," she said enthusiastically.

Melanie did manage to attend the women's circle regularly, and she fit right in. But after a few months I began to notice that her sparkle was fading, and she wasn't participating as much in the conversation. One Sunday when she arrived, she looked drained. When it was her turn to share, big tears welled up in her eyes. "I'm afraid I can't do this job," she whispered. "I'm exhausted, and I've started missing deadlines at work. They just never seem to stop. I push myself out of bed in the morning and try to pretend that everything is normal. But by the time the day is over, all I want to do is get back in bed and play games on my phone."

In California, she told us, she'd liked the long hours and the big paycheck. The stress and deadlines felt motivating. All her colleagues around her were doing basically the same thing, working late into the night, wired on coffee. It just seemed like what you did. But now she was working at home, going into the office only once a week, and sitting in front of a screen or on the phone for at least ten hours a day, including every weekend. As a team leader she was responsible for a dozen people, fielding their phone calls and emails. "If you walked into my home office," Melanie said, trying to laugh, "you'd see a half dozen unfinished cups of coffee and granola bar wrappers all over my desk. I am drowning in work," she said. "I feel like I have nothing left to give—to anyone or anything. I feel numb—not happy, not sad."

I could see that, overworked and not caring for herself, Melanie had fallen out of her Window of Tolerance into hypoarousal. "I can hear how exhausted you are, Melanie, like everything has been taken out of you. When we find ourselves depleted, less interested in things we usually like to do, we lose our joy in life. What you're describing could be seen as a mild level of depression."

"I never thought I could get to this point," Melanie said.

"I can relate to the way you're feeling," Eve responded. "I have pulled a lot of all-nighters myself. Who hasn't?" she smiled, looking around the circle. "So, I recognize burnout. But I've come to realize that when I start going down, something else is also happening. Depression runs in my family, several of us have been diagnosed with it. When I was seventeen, my boyfriend broke up with me right before prom, and I couldn't stop crying for a whole week. Nothing seemed worthwhile. I started feeling like my mother, just wanting to sit on the couch watching television all day. I started having suicidal thoughts around that time. That episode of depression lasted a few weeks, but when it returned during my first year in college, I finally went to see the school counselor and eventually started taking an antidepressant. It made all the difference. That has helped me get through some tough times. I stayed on the meds for a couple of years and then I was able to work with my therapist to get off them. And I wouldn't hesitate to use them again if I needed to."

Annette nodded. "But sometimes I think it's just what's going on in our lives that can get us so depressed," she began. "When my mother died, I fell into a dark time. I had been very close to her. She was my hero. I had been with her every day for the last few weeks of her life and was with her when she took her last breath. During Shiva, the Jewish week of mourning following a death, there were people at the house every day, sitting around looking at photo albums and telling stories. But after that week, I was alone again with a hollow space in my heart, and depression landed. My life felt like a photograph that had all the color taken out of it. Everything seemed gray. All I could do was go to work and come home. I had no appetite for food, no appetite for life. It was one of the hardest times of my life."

As we continued talking, it seemed that most of the women in the group had experienced some level of depression in their lives. The reasons varied but the experience of feeling down from exhaustion, from sadness or grief, from being rejected was familiar. "Any of us may have the blues for a few days," I said, wanting to offer some perspective. "We might feel low when we have given too much of ourselves, or when we experience loss or other unwelcome changes in our life. At those times we might feel dejected, irritable, and unsociable. But if negative self-talk deepens into the kind of feelings Eve mentioned, it might be a sign of a more severe depressive disorder. That's when we might feel a sense of worthlessness or overcome by guilt or shame. We have a hard time doing even simple daily tasks, and we want to withdraw from others.

When that happens to someone, it is important to be on the lookout for any signs that self–harm is being considered. Suicidal thoughts might arise when someone is depressed or in pain, but these are often fleeting with no real intention to act on them. But if such thoughts of escape escalate, that can lead to actual plans for suicide. If anyone you know talks about wanting to harm themselves or wishes that "it would all be over," it is important to ask them directly if they are thinking about taking their life and if they have a plan for how they might do that."

"When we or anyone we know is experiencing severe depression, it is important to be on the lookout for any signs that self–harm is being considered. Suicidal thoughts that arise when someone is depressed or in pain may be fleeting with no real intention to act on them. At those times we want to make sure that person has the support they need to cope with their depression. But it is always important to take it seriously when someone talks about suicide and ask them directly if they are thinking about taking their life and if they have a plan for how they might do that."

"Yes, but wouldn't asking them that question plant the idea of doing it in their mind?" Erin asked with concern.

"No, according to those who work in this field, asking that can save lives. It can give them an opening to talk about what's going on for them. And if you know someone is in danger in this way, it's important to not leave them alone and to step in to get help. You might urge them to call the suicide crisis line, 988, or reach out to mental health or medical professionals. Or you might call that number yourself if you need guidance on what to do."

Ilana had been listening intently as I talked about this, and when I was done, she said, "I know something about this. When Mark left me for another woman, I went into months of depression. I felt devastated and had no idea of how I could get through life. The future looked bleak and empty and unmanageable. One night at two in the morning, I found myself on the floor of my living room sobbing, feeling utterly alone, and for the first time ever the thought of suicide came up in my mind. I got so scared. I really didn't want to die. I just knew that something had to change. I called two friends and asked if they would come over. They held me through the night, and in the morning, they helped me look up the names of some therapists. They're the ones who gave me your number for our women's circle. The support of my friends was what I needed that night, and I started turning my life around."

Being in the depths of despair and losing the wish to live are symptoms of hypoarousal. Often that state can be so consuming and debilitating that we need the support and care of others to help us find our way back into the Window of Tolerance. Even though Ilana recognized that something needed to change, she couldn't get through that dark night alone. I felt grateful that she had reached out to her friends.

Sensing we were all in a tender place, I suggested we do a compassion meditation. I invited the women to come and sit a little closer to each other and close their eyes. "Let yourself notice the echoes of these stories inside yourself and take a few easy breaths." We sat quietly for a couple of minutes. "Now let's open to holding ourselves with compassion. You might want to use the phrase, 'I care about this pain.'" I could sense them settling into the meditation and felt my own heart opening with care for all they had revealed. After a few minutes I asked them to reach out and take the hands of the women sitting next to them. "Let's breathe together as one heart, knowing we all have moments when we feel low and disconnected, and we can hold this unease with compassion and lovingkindness ... And when you feel ready, you can open your mind and heart to others ... to women who, like you, might be feeling exhausted or depressed ... women who have experienced loss ... women who are trying to find their way back to themselves. Expand the warmth of compassion to them, wishing them to be free of suffering. Imagine holding hands with those women and strengthening each other, knowing you are not alone." I saw tears coming down Melanie's face. We closed the meditation by chanting a song we had learned together a few months before: "Courage, sister, you do not walk alone. / We will be with you on your journey home."

As we were nearing the end of the circle, I wanted to send them off with something that would hold them during the month. "When we are exhausted or feel down, it might seem like there is no break in the heavy sad feelings. But when we look carefully, we can notice that even the darkest cloud of depression is not unchanging. There are times when we do feel lighter, less weighed down."

Sandra nodded. "That happens to me when I hear a song I like on the radio, and I find myself singing along. It doesn't mean that what's troubling me goes away, but it does lift me for a minute."

Melanie leaned forward. "If I walk outside late at night after a long day of work and look at the night sky, it reminds me of being on the farm as a child, and that sort of lifts me up. In the summer we used to sleep out on the porch and look up at the stars." As she talked, her face and voice seemed to get a little lighter.

"Those are good examples of ways that can help us find a thread that will lead us out of depression. They can remind us of what we feel like when we're not under that cloud, and even for a moment we remember what we are wanting to return to." I suggested that during the next month everyone make star gazing or listening to a song they like a regular practice. There were lots of smiles in response.

Coming out of depression and returning to a sense of vitality can take some time. We might feel like we are taking steps forward and then find ourselves sliding back. We might see glimmers of possibility and then lose sight of them. But taking even small steps can begin to lift the fog as we find our way back into our Window of Tolerance.

> If you are having suicidal thoughts, wanting to hurt yourself, or feeling in crisis, or if anyone you know is feeling that way, you can call 988 at any time of day or night and receive immediate support. People who are hearing impaired can dial 711 and then 988.

Nurturing Ourselves Back into Balance

At the next gathering of the women's circle, I was glad to see Melanie chatting with some of the others before we sat down. When it was her turn to check in, she told us that looking up at the stars had seemed to open up something inside of her. "Seeing Orion and the Big Dipper was like being with old friends, and looking at all the stars made me feel like I was part of something bigger than my own little life. For a few minutes I forgot about work, I forgot about how exhausted I was feeling. I was just there."

"Yes, when we're feeling down, finding glimmers of aliveness like that can remind us that life is more than being caught in emotional distress." I gestured around the circle. "What happened to the rest of you when you went out to look at the stars?"

Ilana spoke tenderly. "Looking at the stars reminded me of that night when I was so distraught after Mark left. My friends took me outside at some point. It was windy, and clouds were rushing across the sky. Suddenly there was an opening in them, and I could see Venus shining brightly above the horizon and, near it, a crescent moon. I knew that in a few days it would be full. And I got it—things always change, and I could let them. I could change my life."

"Being outdoors like that has always been healing for me," Annette said. "Looking up into the sky made me think of the time after my mother died and I felt so low. I sometimes wondered if that feeling would ever change and if I'd ever be happy again. Once I started taking daily walks in the woods, being among the trees brought me back. And the other night, like Ilana, looking at the stars helped me remember that it's possible to get through hard times."

Eve smiled and said, "I can relate to that. I decided to do what you suggested about listening to a song I like. One came to mind that I had learned when I was part of the choir in college. It was during that difficult time, and joining my voice with others made such a difference in how I felt. This month, singing at home, I didn't hold myself back. Each time I sang, I got louder and bolder," she laughed. "I think singing is my real medicine."

Whether they had looked at the stars or listened to music, everyone had felt joy by choosing to connect to something that lifted their spirits. I suggested that we take a few minutes to practice holding ourselves in those good feelings and then sending out lovingkindness to others. When I rang the bell to end the meditation, everyone looked quietly happy.

"Choosing to do things that nurture us can be another way to offer love to ourselves. Like practicing metta, engaging in activities that gladden our heart can lift us out of difficult thoughts and feelings. Even if you fall back into them, you have had a taste of feeling lighter again. Strengthening wholesome mindstates calls us back from self–abandonment." I suggested that during the next month they keep nurturing themselves with experiences to foster feelings of joy and spaciousness.

"What is one thing you would love to do just for yourself?" I asked them. "Maybe something you haven't done in a long time, something that can help you feel nurtured and cared for."

Eve said she would pick up her violin that had been lying in the closet for months and learn a new Irish tune. Annette, who had a special love for animals, said she would go and pet cats at the animal shelter. A couple of women said they wanted to pull out their old CDs and listen to favorite songs they hadn't heard in years. Ilana said she would dance. Melanie waited until the others were done speaking, and she seemed hesitant as she started talking. "I know what my thing to do would be, but I'm just not sure if I can do it. I have so little time...."

"I can understand how that would be a challenge, Melanie, but can I push you a little? If you knew it was okay to do something for just yourself, what would that be?"

Sitting up a little straighter, she said. "Alright, here it is. I would sit at the corner coffee shop with a large mug of Americano coffee, a spinach–feta pastry, and the *New York Times*. Then I would take out my notebook and write, for a long time, with no interruptions." There were nods of encouragement in the room. Melanie giggled with embarrassment at the positive attention and then said thoughtfully, "Maybe that was what going to church meant for my mother. It was the one time during the week that she could take time for herself. It was a sacred time for her. I think that's what nourished her so she could nourish others."

It turned out that Melanie couldn't wait for a whole month until our next circle to share her story with me. When she called, I could hear the delight in her voice. "I just did it!" she said. On Saturday morning I got out of my pajamas, put on my denim overalls, closed the door behind me, and headed out. I almost felt like skipping. Walking into the café, I smelled the aroma of freshly roasted coffee beans. After placing my order, on my way to my table, I grabbed a free copy of the *Times*. Looking around, I thought to myself: *Not everyone works on a Saturday morning. There are people who do this, and today I am one of them.* I took out my phone and texted the women from our circle, *Arrived!* And then I spent the next hour and a half writing."

Melanie went on to tell me that when she returned home that day, nothing in the house had changed, her to-do list was still as long as it had been before she left, and the laundry had not been put away. There were still as many messages in her inbox, but her heart was lighter, and instead of sinking back under a cloud of depression, she was able to sit down at her desk and start to catch up on the work she had not been able to face the night before.

It would take a few more months after that first joyful morning for Melanie to learn how to sustain a more balanced life. When thoughts came up telling her she was not doing enough at work and she had to put in more hours, she realized she could sit back for a moment, hold herself in lovingkindness and just allow those thoughts to pass. The pause helped her pull out of self-judgment, and she could better consider how to get her work done without abandoning herself. And she began to find ways to care for herself in order to stay within her Window of Tolerance. She faithfully took a lunch break every day, sometimes going for a run in the neighborhood around her office, and once a week she would turn off her computer early and go see a movie, often inviting one of the women from the circle to join her. Every Saturday morning, Melanie continued to take her special time at the coffee shop, and every time she pulled out her notebook to write, it felt like a personal victory.

When we give ourselves permission to nurture ourselves, we return to being grounded and present and able to meet life openly and with spaciousness. Caring for our body and our mind, giving ourselves the time to engage in that which gladdens our heart, is one of the ways we can return to abiding in the Window of Tolerance and greet the world with aliveness, responding to challenges with balance and grace.

Nurturing the Heart

What are some ways in which you have been nurtured in the last few days? You might begin by remembering how the Earth supports you through the air you breathe and the water you drink. Maybe your dog cuddled with you, or a friend offered you some words of appreciation. And how have you nurtured yourself? Perhaps you nurtured your body by riding your bicycle or eating delicious food, nurtured your mind by reading an inspiring book, or nurtured your emotions by listening to beautiful music. Or maybe you sat down to meditate and felt the ease of being present in the moment, or maybe you spent time in prayer. Notice what you feel as you reflect on these ways of being nurtured and allow this fullness of heart to guide and strengthen you.

Turning Back from Trauma

Just before her baby was born, Colleen told us she was going to take a break from therapy and the women's circle to focus on being a mother. I was delighted to get a call from her a couple of months later to tell me that she had given birth to a beautiful boy and named him Galen, which means calm in Greek. She said that having a calm baby had been her dream, but even as an infant, Galen was sensitive to sounds and easily overstimulated. She assured me that she was using mindfulness and lovingkindness to work on her reactivity and to help her stay centered. She said she liked singing the metta phrases as a lullaby to help Galen go to sleep every night. She wanted him to be held by the loving voice she had not grown up with.

After that I didn't hear from her for a long time, and I hoped she was doing well. But one day she called and asked to see me. Galen was around a year old, and when he got upset, he would bite and hit or bang his head against her chest. "Every time he does that, I feel such a strong surge of anger and I want to hit him back. I practice pausing at the about–to–moment, and I have not hit him, but I can barely control the urge to. I'm afraid I'm going to hurt him some day. That is the last thing I would ever want to do." She looked away for a moment, turned back and said, "I don't know how to handle this." As I listened, I remembered her talking about her fear of repeating her mother's behaviors, and my sense was that her strong feelings and impulse to hit stemmed from her own unhealed childhood trauma.

As we have seen in the stories of other women, trauma that has not been addressed and understood can continue to affect us for years after the traumatic event. Unhealed, it can manifest in our bodies as chronic pain and discomfort or, like Megan, feeling disconnected from parts of our body. It can manifest emotionally as anger or anxiety, depression or emotional withdrawal. Or it shows up in behaviors such as hypervigilance, or a strong need to control everyone and everything that might feel like a threat. These symptoms might be the ongoing backdrop of our lives, or they might arise suddenly when something in the present moment triggers a memory of the past.

When we are triggered, we are suddenly overcome by a powerful surge of emotion and our reactions may be out of proportion to the stimulus that brought it on. We are thrown out of our Window of Tolerance into hyper–or hypoarousal, and we want to fight, run away, or collapse. We can be triggered by almost anything—the loud voice of a man or a woman yelling, by sights, sounds, or smells that awaken a memory, or by touch that reminds us of a time when we were not safe. And we can be triggered, like Colleen, when our child's behavior awakens unhealed memories from our early years. We can find ourselves reacting with the intensity of emotion we felt in our own childhood and feel compelled to repeat the hurtful or abusive behaviors we experienced at that time.

As I listened to Colleen talk about her urge to hit Galen, I carefully paid attention to any signs that this might be a dangerous situation for her child. If I thought that this could become uncontrollable anger with the possibility of physical abuse, I would have to take steps to intervene. But over the years of knowing her in the women's group and in therapy, I had seen the sincerity of her intention to heal the anger from her past that had been harming her relationship with Jacob, and so I felt a sense of reassurance that Galen was not in any real danger from her. Colleen was instead experiencing that edge of frustration and exhaustion so many of us have known as parents. Our previous work together and her mindfulness practice had made her well aware of the habit of reaction she could fall into, and I wanted to help her heal some of the source of her pain.

"I can understand how frightening those feelings might be, Colleen," I said. "Let's explore this a little further. Can you tell me more about what you feel when Galen hits or bites you?"

"I suddenly feel light–headed and like my hands are burning. My shoulders, my neck, my arms get so tight. I feel like I'm preparing for a battle. It all happens so fast that I don't even have time to think."

"When such a strong urge like that arises, it might be pointing to a very old hurt that you have not yet been able to heal. I have found that turning to the body with care and sensitivity can be a safe way to explore those feelings. Could we try that?" She nodded and I asked her to bring to mind a time with Galen when he was screaming and crying and hitting her. Colleen closed her eyes. "When an image comes up, stay with it, and let yourself notice what you are feeling in your body."

After a couple of minutes, she said, "I feel that burning sensation in my hands again."

"Stay with that sensation now. Does it bring up any memories or feelings?"

A shudder went through her body. She opened her eyes and looked scared. "I remember my mother gathering all of us around the kitchen table and yelling uncontrollably. Sometimes she'd start hitting us. I was maybe five or six years old. This happened a lot, and I was never sure what I had done wrong. It was terrifying. When she was done, I would run to my room and hide in the closet so she couldn't find me. Sometimes I'd line my dolls up and do the same thing to them. So, when Galen hits me, I feel like I'm back there. I'm scared and angry. Everything feels out of control, and I just want to lash out."

I asked Colleen to stand up and let her body do whatever it needed to do. She got to her feet, her whole body trembling. "I am so angry. How did she dare? I was so little," she said. She stomped around the room and then suddenly, her voice rising, she said, "This is not about Galen. And it sure wasn't about me. But that's what I learned—when you feel overwhelmed, just start yelling, like I do with Jacob. Or start hitting, like I want to do with Galen." Colleen's knees were shaking. She sat down and started sobbing.

After the waves of emotion had passed, I gently said, "Some very old feelings just got stirred up. As we sit here together, see if you can you hold yourself tenderly as you feel the ripples of emotion rising and passing." I watched as her body slowly relaxed and her breath grew easier. After a few minutes, she took a deep breath, blew it out softly, and nodded with a little smile.

"What was that like for you to remember that experience and go through those feelings?" I asked.

"It was intense, and surprising what came up. But it helped to know you were here. I could let those feelings come up without being afraid of getting lost in them."

When traumatic memories break through unexpectedly, it is helpful and often necessary to work with a counselor, a spiritual teacher, or someone who is trustworthy and skilled in healing emotional wounds. Without such support, these emotions may add to our trauma and to the "unbearable aloneness" Diana Fosha, the trauma therapist, talks about. Doing the work in a safe environment supports us in meeting the pain of those overwhelming feelings with wisdom, compassion, and equanimity, allowing them to heal.

As Colleen was getting ready to leave, I encouraged her to be gentle with herself. "It might be good for you to take a short walk before going home, and tonight you might want to send lovingkindness to that little girl who went through such a frightening time. Healing her trauma will help you to not pass it down to Galen. You can also call on the power of pausing at the about-to-moment to help you keep yourself and Galen safe."

The next time we met, Colleen told me that a few days after our session, Galen had a hard day and started hitting again. She said she felt heat rising in her body and her throat tightening, and along with that, a strong impulse to hit him so he would stop hitting her. Somehow right there in the midst of this, she managed to remember the about-to-moment and the possibility of pausing. Pulled between the urge to hit him and her sudden awareness that Galen, her baby, was in pain, Colleen stopped. She took a few deep breaths, and with him still kicking and crying, she put him in the stroller and got them both out the door for a walk. "As I circled the block, Galen began calming down, but I was still fuming. Wave after wave of anger kept moving through me—at him ... at myself ... at my mother. I felt the humiliation and the terror I used to feel when she yelled and hit us. Gradually I started noticing the feeling of my footsteps on the ground, the sound of the passing cars, the leaves on the trees shaking in the wind. The feelings shifted from anger to sadness, and the tears started coming.

"Galen had fallen asleep, and I took him back inside and put him in his bed. I went and stood by the window looking out into the garden and wrapped my arms around my body. My heart was aching. So much pain in all those years of chaos. I stood there until the tears slowed down and the tightness in my throat softened."

After a little while Collen heard Galen crying. She went to his room and gently picked him up. His gaze met hers, and they both smiled. As he snuggled his head into her shoulder, she quietly sang the metta phrases to him. Grateful for not abandoning herself that day, Colleen knew that for both their sakes she was breaking the cycle of trauma.

Over time, as she continued to pay attention to the about-to-moment, Colleen was more able to remain in her Window of Tolerance, even when Galen hit her. When she got triggered and the impulse to react would arise, she increasingly remembered to pause, drop her attention into her body, and allow the waves of emotion to come to completion before she responded. She found that the calmer she was, the easier it was for him to regulate his own body. Together they were learning ways to bring themselves back to center.

> ## When We Are Triggered
>
> The next time you feel a strong sudden surge of emotion arising in you, let yourself pause. Notice what sensations you are feeling in your face, heart, shoulders, abdomen.... What thoughts and emotions are arising? Now bring to mind someone who deeply cares about you—this might be a loving friend, your favorite aunt, your dog or cat. Or you might call upon your wise and compassionate self. Let yourself be gently held by their presence and love as the sensations rise, shift, and change. As the wave of emotion subsides, feel your feet on the floor and take a few deep breaths. Just notice what you are feeling now and honor that. You may want to stay with this process longer or, if you need to, return to it again later. Thank yourself for taking the time to be present in this way.

We all find ourselves out of balance at times. Whether we are highly charged with emotion in hyperarousal or feeling depressed and fatigued in hypoarousal, we lose touch with our wise and compassionate self. As we become aware of the thoughts and emotions that arise when we are lost in reactivity, depression, or trauma, with mindfulness and compassion we can begin to turn back to ourselves. We might notice that we are trying too hard to please others; we might have ignored our need for rest, for exercise, or for intellectual or cultural stimulation. As we listen to our body and recognize that we have lost our emotional balance, we can remember to be gentle with ourselves and pay attention to what we need. When we are overwhelmed by the demands of our daily life, we can pause and ask ourselves if there is anything we can let go of to bring us back into the Window of Tolerance. We no longer have to be "Superwoman" who can do everything but nurture herself.

We can't always change the external circumstances to reduce our stress, but we can change the inner landscape in which they happen. As we cultivate mindfulness, lovingkindness, and compassion, we grow in our ability to hold ourselves with kindness when we have left the Window of Tolerance. We can widen that window by developing wholesome qualities, such as patience and equanimity, to help us stay centered, calm, and spacious in response to the circumstances of our daily life, no matter what they are.

Staying within the Window of Tolerance can be likened to tuning a stringed instrument, such as a guitar or violin. When the string is too tight, the tone is sharp and the string may pop. When the string is too loose, the instrument is lacking in tone. Likewise, if we are caught up in the surges of emotion, we need to relax the tension. If we're feeling blue, we need to find ways to lift our spirits again. Just as a stringed instrument needs to be tuned, we need to tune our inner balance by bringing ourselves back into the Window of Tolerance. Abiding in that spaciousness, we can feel connected to life, come home to ourselves, and love who we are.

Chapter Seven

Befriending Our Lives: Abiding in the Wise and Compassionate Self

The journey from self–abandonment to embracing the wise and compassionate self carries us from the pain of the past to living in the present with a sense of openness and ease. The journey begins with the calling of our heart, the yearning to find a way to be happy with who we are and to live life fully. We discover that we are not at the mercy of habits of self-judgment, self-hatred, and self-doubt but know that we can treat ourselves with kindness. Remembering our innate goodness, we know that we can always turn back to loving and cherishing ourselves. We learn that we can hold ourselves with compassion and care, even in challenging times. Not caught up in painful states of mind, we open to the beauty and abundance of life, and we know we have a place in this world.

Trusting our intention to live and act with wisdom and compassion, we feel more freedom to express our thoughts and our feelings. Knowing that we are worthy of love, we feel more freedom to acknowledge our needs and to ask for support. In touch with our concerns for justice and the welfare of the planet, we feel more freedom to fully engage in compassionate action. And less bound by social conditioning and expectations, we feel more freedom to be who we are. As we respond to the calling of our heart, we are more willing to take risks, try new paths, form new relationships, heal difficult mindstates, and open to the adventures of life.

And yet, as we know, even as we become more deeply aligned with our wise and compassionate self, life does not always give us what we want. Sometimes, no matter what we do or how hard we try, we cannot make our dreams come true. What we want doesn't happen, or what we don't want happens. Life keeps moving through us like a river, some days calm and some days turbulent, and we are constantly navigating the truth of impermanence that the Buddha talked about. One day we may be feeling showered with the gifts of life—everything lining up just the way we want it—and suddenly circumstances change. Maybe you had been acting in a theater show, feeling happy and fulfilled, and then closing night arrived, the curtain came down, and suddenly have you lost your community, your avenue of creative expression, the nightly accolades and appreciation for your role. Maybe you had been enjoying financial security until a recession hit and your investments disappeared. Or maybe, after many years of companionship and a friendship that was core to your life, your marriage has come to an end. For all of us, there are times when the unexpected happens—illness, accidents, bad news—and what we had counted on to define our life has changed.

In moments like this, we may feel sad, frustrated, or angry for not getting what we want or for losing what we had. We may feel disappointed, confused, or guilty, wondering if we could have done anything differently to change the outcome. We may feel that we have lost our identity and don't know who we are, feeling we are on shaky ground with nothing to rely on. How do we not abandon ourselves when life does not align with our dreams and aspirations? How do we hold ourselves with wisdom, love, and kindness even in the midst of unwanted change?

I found myself facing these questions when my life brought me to a significant turning point. When Ian and I got married, and then when Tamar and Noa were born, so many of my wishes had been fulfilled. And yet, despite all these blessings, something in my heart continued to long for the place I still called home—Israel. I had left there as a young person to follow the longing that led me to India and then to living in the United States to deepen my meditation practice. But part of me had continued to believe that when I had children, I would raise them "back home," close to my parents and siblings. Each time I visited Israel, something inside me felt deeply in place. And upon returning to Ithaca, there was always a whisper in my mind: *This is not my home, I don't belong here. Life will really begin when I move back to Israel. Then I will be happy.*

I longed to sit around the table in my parents' narrow dining room, talking about my day as I ate a bowl of my mother's soup, to spend relaxing hours with my old friends, watching our children grow up together. I missed speaking Hebrew, seeing my favorite Israeli musicians, and eating falafel in soft pita bread from the local stand up the road. And all my being wanted to be involved in Israel–Palestine peace activism. No matter how much I tried to talk myself out of these feelings or think my way out of them, the longing in my heart was not going away.

So, when Tamar and Noa were nine and six, Ian and I packed up the house and moved across the ocean to Israel. My wish to have the family we had created near my family of origin was happily fulfilled. My mother made us delicious meals when we visited, and we spent hours talking around the table. She shared songs and riddles with the girls, and my father showed them how to do things, like making a kite or rebinding a favorite book. We shared holiday celebrations and went for long walks on the beach. At last we were in each other's lives. My dream had come true.

Of course, there were a few challenges with settling into our new home, and a new community, and the political climate was not simple. But overall I loved once again being held in the unique cultural matrix of Israel—the quietude that comes over the streets as people get ready for Shabbat on a Friday afternoon; the bells ringing out from the churches in the old city of Jerusalem; and the muezzin chanting the call to prayer at the nearby mosque. I soaked in the feeling of the land, the deep silence of the desert, and the beauty of wildflowers blooming in the oak forest near our home. These familiar experiences resonated with childhood memories held in my body and in my heart. When I participated in gatherings of Israeli and Palestinian peace activists, I felt like I had found kindred spirits and that even our small steps were moving us closer to a sustainable way of living together in this land. By the end of the first year there, I had found my place and doors had begun to open. My life felt meaningful. I had responded to the calling of my heart and my deep yearning had been answered.

But I wasn't the only one in my family with a longing for "home." Toward the end of our second year in Israel, it became clear that Ian and our daughters wanted to return to Ithaca. Ian's mom was aging, and he wanted to be close to her, and the girls longed for the familiarity of their life in the States. I felt torn between the vision I'd held for my life and my unquestioned commitment to Ian and the girls, but there was only one answer—we were going home to Ithaca.

When life does not give us what we want, how do we continue to befriend ourselves? How do we honor the longings of our heart without clinging to them being fulfilled in a particular way? When life does not align with our desires, how do we find peace in being with things as they are? The Buddha taught that happiness is possible even when things don't go the way we expect them to. As we continue to turn back to ourselves, listening to our heart, we learn how to arrive in the moment, to befriend our life as it is, and to let our wise and compassionate self bring us home.

From the Wanting Mind to the Longing Heart

Wanting is an inescapable part of our lives. It moves us from place to place, it is the force behind our choices and actions, and it motivates our creative endeavors. It is how we get our needs met and what makes us reach out for relief from pain. We want to be happy and healthy, we want a meaningful life, and we want to end suffering in the world. Wanting our dreams to be fulfilled and wanting to be happy are not wrong. But when we get attached to getting our desires met in a certain way, when we hold onto an idea of how our life should unfold, that clinging leads to suffering. Caught in the "wanting mind," we believe that our happiness depends on having what we don't have. "If only I had … this relationship, this house, this job … then I would be happy."

The Buddha taught that the antidote to the pain of wanting is letting go—opening the tight fist that is holding onto life being "our way." This does not mean that we endure abusive situations without taking action. It does not mean depriving ourselves of pleasure or ignoring our physical and emotional needs. Rather, it is about freeing ourselves from believing that we can be happy only if our life unfolds in a particular way. Letting go allows us to bring our attention back to our experience in the moment and, in that intimate relationship, discover what life is offering.

But sometimes, even when we're willing and trying to let go, wanting thoughts keep arising in our mind and we cannot get them to stop. At those times, especially when we know we can't get what we want, how do we not abandon ourselves but instead let our wanting lead us to the deeper longing of our heart? This was what I had to discover when my desire to live in Israel was not fulfilled.

When we arrived back in the United States, our first stop was to visit Ian's mother Elsa in her apartment. We parked the car and the girls dashed into the building and ran down the long hallway to catch the elevator up. Granny was there to welcome us at her door with a warm hug, her eyes slightly teary. Seeing her, I remembered why we had returned. She, too, had soup for us and some fruit to take for the road. After a few hours of lively conversation, we continued on to Ithaca. As we drove down the hill into town, I found myself joining the others as we screamed with excitement. This too felt like home.

After all the commotion of settling in and the girls going back to school, reality struck and I landed hard. Even though I had made the decision to return, I had left behind a world I loved. I missed some of the small daily things we did in our town in Israel, like visiting Samir, the handsome butcher with his high cheekbones, and the Friday morning walks on the rocky beaches with Ian. And, of course, my mom and dad. As much as I wanted to, I couldn't shrink the ocean to bring the two countries closer together. I couldn't be in two places at once. Ian and the girls were getting back into their lives, but I was adrift, no longer sure who I was or what my life purpose could be in this place that did not fully feel like home.

Grief arrived, and my heart felt heavy as I sank into depression. Through that veil nothing felt meaningful. I remember one day setting out to buy some vegetables at the small farmers market downtown. As I approached the line of stalls, I could see the farmers chatting with customers over their freshly picked produce, a sight that would typically make me happy. But that day I couldn't connect with any of the beauty in it. Instead, my mind went into judgment. *I don't know these people, and what they are doing is meaningless. There is nothing more important than working for peace in the Middle East. That's where I should be.* I turned around and left, my heart aching with longing to have what I didn't have.

All of us have had moments when the circumstances of our lives have changed in unexpected and undesirable ways. Losing some part of our life or losing a vision of what we would like it to be can feel like a kind of death. We may begin to question who we are and what our life is about. We might try to resist the loss, fight it, not want to accept it. We might feel deeply sad or depressed. We might feel bereft of our connection to our wise and compassionate self, unable to even remember what our heart is most longing for. Each change is a loss of who we used to be, a loss of our sense of who we are, and it is asking us to step into a new "me," someone we do not yet know. We have lost who we once were and have not yet discovered who we have become.

Unable to find my way out of depression, I got in touch with Pam, a therapist I knew and trusted. In her presence, I let myself open to the longing I felt for my family and my friends in Israel, my yearning for the land, the air, the unique smells. In one of our sessions, an image arose in my mind of an olive tree and a fig tree with a fresh vine creeping over them.

"That reminds me of the verse from the bible," Pam said. "*And each person will sit beneath his own grapevine and under his own fig tree and no one will make them afraid.* What do those figs and vines mean to you?"

Images I loved of the Jerusalem Hills flooded my mind. With tears rolling down my face, I told her about visiting my sister's kibbutz, going for walks in the late afternoon, picking sweet figs and grapes off the vine. That felt like home. Some of those olive trees we saw had been there for hundreds of years, some planted by Palestinian farmers. "They loved the land the way I do, and maybe some of the sadness I'm feeling is also for that," I said.

I spent several sessions with Pam, allowing waves of grief for everything I had left behind to move through me. Lines from a poem by John O'Donohue, the Irish mystic and teacher of Celtic spirituality, guided me: "May you have the wisdom to enter generously into your own unease / to discover the new direction your longing wants you to take." I entered into the unease and discomfort of not knowing what my life was about now, allowing the longing to show me the way. I knew that accepting my life and opening to its unique fullness was the only pathway I could follow. But *what would it actually mean to accept my life as it was? And if I accepted my life, would I be happy then?*

Each time grief arose in my heart again, I would gently bring my attention to it and mindfully breathe into the sensation. I began to see that if I entered those feelings with openness and care, some movement and change would occur. Reciting the metta and compassion phrases also brought ease and some relief. Sometimes I cried, many days I went for walks in the woods near my house, and almost every day I called my mother. Being kind to myself, holding myself with loving awareness, and receiving the love of others allowed me to be in the unease without getting lost in it.

I started to ask myself what it was that I was really longing for. What was my heart calling for at this time of my life? Just as following that yearning years before had changed my life and brought me home to myself in a new way, could I trust again that there was something on the other side of this feeling? I was beginning to recognize that beneath the wanting to have the experiences and people and activities that Israel meant to me was a deeper longing, the calling of my heart to feel at home within myself, to find a sense of ease, joy, and connection in my life as it was now. Something in me began to soften and open. The fist that had been holding tight to a memory of the past, an idea of how things should be, was slowly opening to life as it was in that moment, opening to the new direction my longing wanted to take me.

This Is It: Welcoming the Gifts of Life

One early morning a few months after our return to Ithaca, I was riding my bicycle along the fields close to my house. It was an exquisite summer morning. Soft sunlight was reaching down through the breaks in the clouds. The fields were lush and green, and young plants swayed in the gentle breeze. I was enjoying the feeling of my body moving through space, the cool breeze on my face, my muscles working hard as my feet pushed on the pedals. In the midst of that delight, a thought crossed my mind: *This is it. This is my life. That is my house I see in the distance, and these are the fields I see when I walk our dog every day.*

This is it slowly penetrated my being. *This is my life, and it includes living here in Ithaca, away from my parents. This is my life, and it includes going back and forth between being mindful and being absent-minded, sometimes centered and sometimes reactive. This is my life, and it sometimes includes backaches, depression, and anxiety. This is my life, and it includes living in a house that is usually not as tidy as I think it should be or wish it would be. This is it. This is my life.*

As I took in the panorama of clouds hovering on the horizon in soft shades of white and gray, my mind kept revealing the truth of this present moment. *This is it* meant having a family I love and that loves me. *This is it* meant living in a progressive town and being part of a community that shared my values. *This is it* meant having good health that allowed me to be engaged in my life with vitality and joy. *This is it* also meant having opportunities to study the Dharma and share it with others. Reflecting on the blessings of my life, my heart filled with gratitude. For a moment, there was an absence of struggle, and a feeling of surrender arose. Being present, right here in this life, with all its beauty and its challenges, was a source of happiness. My longing for my parents had not gone away, my backaches had not disappeared, but they too were part of my life. I didn't need to deny or push any of it away.

When I arrived home and got off my bicycle, I stood there for a while, opening to this new feeling of embracing my life. This feeling of love and acceptance was not dependent on getting everything right, on my being perfect, on finding solutions to every problem. It was a way of befriending all of who I was now and not abandoning myself because circumstances had changed. I felt showered with metta. Then I carefully leaned my bicycle against the wall of the garage and stepped into the house.

That feeling of being present and blessed in the moment went with me throughout that day. It was there as I gathered up my gardening tools and carried them out to the vegetable beds. It was there as I felt the earth on my fingers when I planted new seedlings of tomato and kale for the next season. Later, sitting on the porch drinking tea, listening to the birds, feeling the tightness in my back, I felt present for my life in a new way, not asking it to be different, welcoming it as it was. Gratitude arose as the natural response of my heart to being open and receptive to life, right now.

Gratitude arises naturally when we pay close attention to the gifts of life and we allow ourselves to be touched by them. As we turn back and befriend ourselves, becoming more comfortable and at ease with who we are, we soften and allow in these gifts. We can cultivate this capacity to feel gratitude by choosing what to focus on in our daily life. Thich Nhat Hanh, the Vietnamese meditation master, writes "To be in touch with the wonderful things in the world—to be able to smile, to be able to enjoy the blue sky, the sunshine, the presence of each other, I think that is the first thing we have to practice."

We can practice shifting our attention to what gladdens our heart. This is not to deny our suffering but also not to deny the goodness in our lives. One of my role models for this is Elsa, my mother-in-law. In the last year or two of her life, as she was losing many of her capacities, the sharp edge that we had experienced as judgment, began to soften and she started paying more attention to what was good in her life. She enjoyed walking around her building in the retirement community, watching sailboats on the lake beyond her window, seeing chipmunks and squirrels scamper around the front lawn. No longer able to get to Lincoln Center in New York for a concert or win a game of Scrabble or read a good novel, she was grateful for the small gifts of life right in front of her. Appreciating such moments cultivates an uplifting way of being in the world.

At one of our monthly gatherings, I asked the women in our circle to share some of the small gifts of life they were grateful for. Ilana was grateful for dancing again with a group of people after the Covid restrictions were lifted. She appreciated the feeling of her body spinning and joining in the excitement of dancers being together. Annette was grateful to get a good night's sleep after several nights of insomnia. She felt happy, her mind was clear, and her body felt energized again. And

Erin told us about the comfort she felt when her dog came up to her and put her paw in her lap when she was crying, and even in the midst of pain, she could still feel gratitude for this gesture of caring.

Even when we find ourselves pulled into judgment or anger, when we find ourselves complaining or resentful about our lot in life, we can still remember that there is something to be grateful for and let ourselves reach out for that. I have learned to pause in the midst of these mind-states to pause and let myself choose a way through. One late afternoon, at the end of a long day, I returned home from work tired and feeling irritated. Nothing felt right. To use one of our family expressions, I was "scanning negative." All I could see was what needed to be attended to in the house, what Ian and the girls had done wrong—or hadn't done at all. I knew I needed to find a way back. I asked Noa, who was in high school at the time, if she would go boating with me. Despite my cranky mood, she happily agreed.

Just seeing the lake from the car, my difficult feelings began to lift. I stretched my arms above my head and released a big yawn. As we settled into our kayaks, my body began to relax. The boats swayed from side to side until they balanced, and we slowly moved forward in silence onto the open water. The sun was setting and the soft light shining on the ripples made by the evening breeze reflected ever–changing shades of gold, blue, and black. I could feel my heart beginning to expand, my breath deepening. I listened to the sound of the boats softly gliding forward. From time to time they bumped into each other, and we gently pushed them apart and moved onward. When darkness fell, we turned back. A great blue heron flew by. Back on shore, we quietly carried the kayaks back to their racks. No longer overcome by agitation, I saw that the evening was full of wonder, and I felt a deep appreciation for being alive. Slowing down, allowing the stress hormones to drain out of my body, and surrounding myself with beauty had allowed gratitude to arise again.

Gratitude deepens each time we meet a moment of beauty with an open heart, knowing it is fleeting—being present with a flower, knowing that it will wither; being present with a child who will grow up and leave home; being present for a moment of joy that will fade. Awareness of the passing of life, the truth of all things changing, nothing to hold onto, fills our life with gratitude for this moment.

A few years ago, I received a phone call from my sister Yael who told me that our father, eighty-six years old, was not doing well. He had dreamed about death for several nights in a row and was plagued by anxiety, feeling that death was knocking on his door. After a few days of deliberation, I decided to fly over and spend time with him. During this visit, I gave myself the gift of being present with my parents without distractions.

My father, who was a lover of the written word, had a special place in his heart for the poetry of Robert Frost. In his study I found the tattered volume of poems we used to read together when I was growing up. I pulled it off the shelf and brought it to the living room. I moved the small stool closer to my father's chair and handed the book to him along with his glasses. He opened it with reverence.

"Let's see," he said, paging through to choose a poem.

I asked if we could read "After Apple Picking," a favorite of mine. I watched him as he slowly turned the pages until he found the right one, stroked it flat with his hand, and began to read. When he got to the lines "... there may be two or three / Apples I didn't pick upon some bough. / But I am done with apple-picking now," he smiled. "No more apple picking for me," he said. "These bones are too tired." We laughed together, despite the wistfulness in his words. We took turns reading other poems until he got tired and said with a smile, "I think that's enough for today," and we both went off to bed. I was filled with gratitude for the preciousness of those moments.

The day before I left to return home, I walked on the beach with my mother, talking about the classes she was taking, about aging, and about my life back in Ithaca. Then I jumped in the salty water and took in the feeling of being tossed by the waves, remembering the total presence I felt as a child, open to life and fully in it. On my last evening there, my father said, "Dalya'le, you can go home now and be with your children, where you belong. I'm doing fine, you don't have to worry. Come again when you can."

Being with my parents with as much presence as I could bring to each moment nurtured all of our hearts. *This is it* was being with them, not knowing if this would be the last visit with my father but knowing that he was there and I was there with him. And when I arrived in Ithaca, *This is it* meant being back home fully present with Ian and the girls. Rather than feeling a dichotomy between my "real life" and a life I was longing for, I felt a continuum of present moments, strung together like a string of pearls, each moment equally precious, each moment shining. Each moment an opportunity for gratitude.

Opening Our Heart to the World

When we have opened our heart to ourselves with lovingkindness and compassion, we naturally open it to the world. We see a family of deer grazing in the meadow near our house, and our heart thrills. We see the first daffodils bloom in our garden, and our heart expands with joy. We meet a friend we haven't seen for a long time, and we feel a rush of love. When love flows through us, we open to the immeasurable number of living beings we share this world with, remembering that we all without exception wish to be happy, we all wish to be free of suffering and live with ease. And yet this very awareness faces us with the immensity of pain in the world and our heart asks what we can do to heal it.

This question has been with me since that night when I was a teenager and watched the movie about the Vietnam War. My mother sat with me on the edge of my bed, helping hold my tears as I faced the truth of not knowing what I could do in response to the suffering I had seen. Later, when I traveled in India and had the opportunity to meet with Mother Theresa for a few minutes in Kolkata, I began to get a clue. She and I talked on the sunny balcony of the convent where she was staying. In answer to my question, "What should I do to help the world?" she said, "Go back home and help there." This is what we each are called to do, to relieve suffering wherever we are "home" and in whatever way we can. Several years later, a workshop with Joanna Macy, activist, eco-philosopher, and founder of the Work that Reconnects, helped me articulate my desire to be involved in peace work. I left that event with an image of holding planet Earth in the palm of my hand.

There is no one right way to respond to the pain of the world. It might be that your work is to heal the pain in your own heart, and that in itself may be enough. You might have just enough energy to be present for one friend or one family member who could use your support. And that will be enough. You might grow vegetables in your back yard, create art, or teach in a school. If you are so inclined, you might want to be out on the streets protesting injustice or canvasing before election days, or you might participate in town meetings. When our heart is open and we feel the pain of the world, we can listen to our deepest wisdom and hear what we are called to do.

I have been inspired by Howard Thurman, twentieth-century American philosopher, theologian, mystic, and civil rights leader, who said, "Don't ask yourself what the world needs. Ask yourself what makes you come alive, and go do that, because what the world needs is people who have come alive." Thurman's words invite us to honor and celebrate our aliveness, to bring joy and zest for life into our inquiry, trusting that from that place we will find a way for our compassionate heart to manifest in the world.

Reaping the Fruits of the Practice

Noa and I were standing on a small observation tower at Poon Hill, a hill station in the Himalayas, 10,000 feet above sea level. We had spent the past three weeks tracing the footsteps of my long-ago journey in India. We'd made our way to Bodh Gaya, back to the Bodhi tree and the Thai temple where I participated in my first meditation retreat. Now in Nepal, we had climbed to this summit overlooking the Annapurna and Dhaulagiri mountain ranges to watch the sunrise. Awestruck by the majesty of the mountains, we found ourselves chanting the prayers we sing at Yom Kippur services as we recommit ourselves to goodness and to recalling our responsibility to the world. The ancient Aramaic song, "Avinu Malkeinu," was invoking a vast love to protect and guide us. The modern hymn, "Return Again" was inviting us to "Return to who you are, return to what you are, return to where you are, born and reborn again." This returning is what I had been doing again and again in my life, in the moments of each day and each time I turned back to myself, opening to a new life.

Turning back to ourselves is the path to our aliveness, to being awake and aware, and fully engaged in our lives. While we may feel this aliveness on top of a mountain or walking on the beach, when we sing or dance, when we are deep in conversation or in meditation, that aliveness is always inside us. Turning back to ourselves opens us to that vitality. The practices we dedicate ourselves to yield that harvest.

In one of our circles, I asked the women if they could put into words the fruit of their years of practice. Ilana said that when she feels overwhelmed and recognizes that something is "off," she has a toolbox she can reach into with practices that help her come back to center. The meditation that used to feel like an esoteric concept to her is now part of her life and something she can turn to at any time.

Eve described her journey as weaving together two threads of connection—one, her deepening connection to herself, and the other,

her connection to others. The more connected she feels to herself, the more connected she feels to the world.

Erin said that lovingkindness and self-acceptance feel to her like a familiar place, a comfortable room she has now visited many times, and she knows how to find her way back there when she is gone too long.

Annette was grateful for learning how to be kind to herself. When she practices mindfulness of her breath, if her mind wanders, she can gently remind herself to bring her attention back to the moment. For her, this is a metaphor for how to live life.

And Colleen spoke about her growing ability to be with waves of fear, physical pain, or rage as they arise, remembering to pause and say to herself, "This too will pass, I can be with it."

As we all know, even when we have turned back to ourselves, there will still be days when we might again be flooded by self-judgment, self-hatred, and self-doubt. There will be times when we feel lonely, rejected, and unworthy. There will be moments when we will get lost in anger, jealousy, or fear. But each time we return to our wise and compassionate self, we can see these difficult mindstates for what they are, not identifying with them and not believing them to be true.

Once we have awakened to our innate goodness and our sense of belonging, we never completely forget that we have a place in the world. Once we have found our way into the embrace of lovingkindness and compassion, we know that this is where we feel at home, and we always know we are worthy of love and care. Once we have tasted the sweetness of being kind to ourselves, we realize we don't want to treat ourselves any other way. No matter how many times we need to turn back again—and again—once we have found our way there, we know how to get back home.

We each have been called to this journey back to ourselves, and we have followed it through the ripples of our life story and into that deeper part of ourselves that is unharmed, our wise and compassionate self that holds the pearl of love within us. We discover new depths of happiness and inner peace, and as lovingkindness blossoms in our heart, we welcome it home. Being touched by lovingkindness can feel like being touched by the divine, like a door has opened to the mystery. We get glimmers of a boundless love that is all–embracing, not constrained by time or place. We experience ourselves as a wave in the ocean, arising from the ocean, returning to the ocean, always part of it, never separate.

Our journey continues as we each step into the unknown and walk the path back to ourselves, alone and together. My wish and prayer are that this work of turning back to yourself and returning to abide in your wise and compassionate self will benefit you and ripple out into the world in ever–widening circles.

> May you be happy, peaceful, healthy,
> and at home within yourself.
>
> May you remember your innate goodness and
> your belonging on this Earth.
>
> May wisdom, compassion, and lovingkindness lead you
> and support you on your way.
>
> May your practice be of benefit to all living beings.

Acknowledgments

I see this book as a collaborative project. It came into being thanks to my editor, teachers, family, and friends who supported me in making this book a reality. To all of you, I offer my gratitude.

To my editor Shoshana Alexander for the deepest possible exploration of self-abandonment and the path back to ourselves. Through countless drafts and hours of work together, we wrestled with the ideas and explored the interface of teaching from the Theravada Buddhism tradition, experiential psychotherapy, and feminist thinking. Shoshana taught me how to pay attention to every word, to be intentional in each sentence, and to stay committed to clarity. She taught me how to craft stories, and how to weave them together with the dharma (Buddhist teachings), and she added her touch of beauty to each page. To you, Shoshana, I am deeply grateful.

I offer my gratitude to Bridget Meeds, my student and friend, who suggested I write this book. She edited what I called the "original manuscript" and kept urging me to bring the book to fruition. Thank you, Bridget, for your vision and encouragement, your wisdom, and your love.

To friends and family who read and edited multiple drafts. Thank you for your thoughtful comments and questions and for reminding me that the journey was worthwhile. To Ian Shapiro, Tamar Shapiro-Tamir, Mihal Ronen, Robyn Bem, and Shira Nayman, thank you for your keen eyes, especially in the final days of the work. And to the book designer, Bostjan Lisec, for his skill and artistry.

To my parents, Adele and Yehuda Tamir, who loved me unconditionally and gave me the foundation for loving myself. They believed in me and trusted me when I set off on my life journey, and they planted in me the courage to manifest my dreams. To my siblings, Ilan and Yael, for the safety net they have always been for me.

To Ian, my husband, who has been supporting my spiritual path since the moment we met. He has been my backwind for these years of writing, allowing me time and space to do the work. This book would not have come to completion without his support.

To our daughters for teaching me about joy, resilience, confidence, and creativity, for modeling the possibility of living a full unhindered life in an ever-changing world, for offering the perspective of the LGBTQ community, and for calling me out on my blind spots. I'm grateful for their patience and their love.

Special thanks to my teacher and mentor James Baraz, who believed in me and encouraged me to be a vehicle for the truth. A heartfelt gratitude to my mentor and therapist Carol Drexler, who taught me how to turn back to myself and hold myself in kindness.

To my meditation teachers in the Insight Meditation tradition: Joseph Goldstein, Sharon Salzberg, Fred Von Allmen, Christopher Titmuss, Christina Feldman, Michel McDonald, Larry Rosenberg, Narayan Helen Liebenson, Rodney Smith. To my teachers in the Tibetan tradition Anne C. Klein (Lama Rigzin Drolma,) and Harvey Aronson (Lama Namgyal Dorje).

To my psychotherapy teachers: Diana Fosha, Peter Levine, Richard Schwarz, Janina Fisher, Linda Graham, and to Jalaja Bonheim for teaching me the art and skill of leading women's circles.

To Joanna Macy for extending the invitation to participate in the healing of the world. To Bill Plotkin for his understanding of human development and offering the possibility of living an eco-centric life.

To all the women who have been walking the path back to themselves, for your courage and wisdom, for your sincere practice, and for your contribution to creating a safe, sustainable, and just world.

Resources

1. Kearney-Cooke, Ann, and Tieger, Diana. "Body Image Disturbance and the Development of Eating Disorders." *The Wiley Handbook of Eating Disorders*, edited by Linda Smolak and Michael P Levine, Wiley & Sons, Inc., 2015, pp. 283–296.
2. Gardner, Christopher. "Study: People with Eating Disorders Infrequently Seek Help for Symptoms." *Yale School of Medicine*. July 18, 2019.
3. *The Social and Economic Cost of Eating Disorders in the United States of America: A Report for the Strategic Training Initiative for the Prevention of Eating Disorders and the Academy for Eating Disorders*. Deloitte Access Economics, June 2020.
4. Arcelus, Jon, Mitchell, Alex J., Wales, Jackie, and Nielsen, Søren. "Mortality Rates in Patients with Anorexia Nervosa and Other Eating Disorders: A Meta–analysis of 36 Studies." *Archives of General Psychiatry*. 2011.

Recommended Reading

Baraz, James and Shoshana Alexander. *Awakening Joy: 10 Steps to True Happiness.* Parallx Press. 2012.

Brach, Tara. *Radical Acceptance: Embracing Your Life with The Heart of a Buddha.* Batman, 2003.

Bonheim, Jalaja. *The Magic of Circlework: The Practice Women Around the World are Using to Heal Themselves.* Meeting in Sacred Places. 2018.

Brown, Brene. *The Gifts of Imperfection: Let Go of Who You Think You're Supposed to Be and Embrace Who You Are.* Hazelden Publications, 2010.

Chodron, Pema. *When All Things Fall Apart: Heart Advice for difficult times.* Shambala Publications, 1997.

Chodron, Pame. Welcoming the Unwelcome: Wholehearted Living in a Brokenhearted World. Shambala publications, 2019.

Fisher, Janina. *Healing the Fragmented Selves of Trauma Survivors: Overcoming Internal Self Alienation.* Routledge, 2017.

Fosha, Diana. *Undoing Aloneness and the Transformation of Suffering Into Flourishing: AEDP 2.0.* American Psychology Association, 2021.

Graham, Linda. Bouncing Back: Rewiring Your Brian for Maximum Resilience And Well Being. New World Library, 2013.

Levine, Peter. *In An Unspoken Voice: How the Body Releases Trauma and Restores Goodness.* North Atlantic Books, 2010.

Levine, Peter. *Walking The Tiger: Healing Trauma.* North Atlantic Books, 1997.

Liebenson, *Narayan. The Magnanimous Heart. Compassion and Love, Loss and Grief, Joy and Liberation.* Wisdom Publications, 2018.

Macy, Joanna, Young, Molly. Coming Back to Life: Practices to Reconnect Our Lives, Our World. New Society Publishers, Revised ed. 2014,

Neff, Kristen. *Self-Compassion. The Proven Power of Being Kind to Yourself.* William Morrow, 2011.

Pinkola Estes, Clarissa. *Women Who Run With the Wolves: Myths and Stories of the Wild Woman Archetype.* Ballantine Books, 1992.

Plotkin, Bill. Nature and the Human Soul: Cultivating Wholeness and Community in a Fragmented World. New World Library, 2008. 1998.

Salzberg, Sharon. *Lovingkindness: The Revolutionary Art of Happiness.* Shambala Publications, 1995.

Salzberg, Sharon. *Faith: Trusting Your Own Deepest Experience.* Riverhead Books, 2003.

Schwartz, Richard. *No bad Parts. Healing Trauma and Restoring Wholeness with Internal Family Systems.* Sounds True, 2021.

Siegel, Daniel. *Mindsight: The New Science of Personal Transformation.* Bantam Books, 2010.

Smith, Rodney. *Awakening: A Paradigm Shift of the Heart.* Shambala Publication, Inc, 2014.

About the Author

Dalya Tamir's path of transformation began in the small village of Bodh Gaya, India, in 1983, where she participated in a ten-day silent meditation retreat. Since then, many years of meditation practice and study of Buddhist teachings taught her about the potential we all have to liberate our hearts from suffering. Her training in social work exposed her to teachings about systems of oppression and ways large systems affect the individual. This understanding strengthened her commitment to social justice, especially in the areas of women's liberation and peace building.

Dalya has been facilitating meditation circles for women in Ithaca NY and in Israel since 2002. During a two-year sabbatical in Israel, she led meditation and dialogue groups for Israeli Jews and Palestinians. She has worked as a psychotherapist in community mental health settings as well as in private practice. Dalya aspires to create safe spaces for people to access their innate wisdom and compassion.

Printed in the USA
CPSIA information can be obtained
at www.ICGtesting.com
CBHW040358140424
6791CB00008B/17